Dr Bruce

Wind of Chance

The Pentland Press Ltd.
Edinburgh Cambridge Durham

© M. M. Nicol, 1991

First published in 1991 by
The Pentland Press Ltd.
Brockerscliffe
Witton Le Wear
Co. Durham

All rights reserved. No part of this publication may be reproduced, stored in a retrieval system, or transmitted in any form or by any means, mechanical, photocopying, recording or otherwise, without the written permission of the publisher.

ISBN 0 946270 98 8

Typeset by Polyprint,
48 Pleasance, Edinburgh EH8 9TJ

Printed and bound in Britain by
Polyprint, 48 Pleasance, Edinburgh EH8 9TJ

Cover design by Geoff Hobbs

Contents

		Page
List of Publications		vii
List of Illustrations		xii
Foreword		xiii
Obituary		xv
Chapter 1	Family Background	1
Chapter 2	Youth and Medical Studies	10
Chapter 3	Practising as a Doctor	24
Chapter 4	Medical Service in India	55
Chapter 5	Early Service in Nigeria	66
Chapter 6	Family Interlude	94
Chapter 7	The Delta Province	106
Chapter 8	Return to Warri	120
Chapter 9	Back to Kaduna	130
Chapter 10	Developing Personal Roots in England	166

List of Publications

1939 Nicol, B.M. and Lyall, A., *Lancet*, i, 3. "The gastric secretions during pathological hypochloraemia".
1939 Lyall, A. and Nicol, B.M., *J. Physiol. 96*, 21. "The gastric secretions in experimental hypochloraemia".
1939 Nicol, B.M., *Lancet*, ii, 881. "The control of gastric acidity in peptic ulcer" *9*, 1.
1940 Nicol, B.M., *Quarterly J. Med.* "The renal changes in alkalosis".
1941 Nicol, B.M., *Brit. Med. J.*, ii, 780. "The geographical distribution of gastric and peptic ulcer in the British Isles, with notes on the aetiology of peptic ulcer".
1942 Nicol, B.M., *Lancet*, i, 466. "Peptic Ulceration; the results of modern treatment".
1949 Nicol, B.M., *Brit. J. Nutr., 3*, 25. "Nutrition of Nigerian Peasant Farmers, with special reference to the effects of Vitamin A and Riboflavine deficiency".
1952 Nicol, B.M., *Brit. J. Nutr., 6*, 34. "The Nutrition of Nigerian Peasant Farmers, with special reference to the effects of deficiencies of the Vitamin B complex, Vitamin A and animal protein".
1953 Nicol, B.M., *Brit. Med. J.*, ii, 177. "The use and effectiveness of antimalarial drugs".
1953 Nicol, B.M., *West African Med. J., 2*, 3. "Food, Population and Health in West Africa".
1953 Nicol, B.M., Proc. Nutr. Soc., 12, 66. "Protein in the Diet of the Isoko Tribe of the Niger Delta".
1953 Nicol, B.M., *Am. J. Clin. Nutr., 1*, 364. "Tribal Nutrition and Health in Nigeria".
1954 Nicol, B.M., Ann. New York Acad. Sci., *57*, 764. "The question of the relative importance of protein and labile methyl in the development of fatty liver and cirrhosis in man".
1955 Mann, G..V, Nicoll, B.M. and Stare, F.J., *Brit. Med. J.*, ii, 1008. "The beta-lipoprotein and cholesterol concentration in sera of Nigerians".

LIST OF PUBLICATIONS

1955 Nicol, B.M., "Feeding Nigeria", Federal Information Service, Nigeria.
1956 Nicol, B.M., *West African Med. J.*, 5, 157. "An evaluation of the specific gravity method for estimating the haemoglobin, packed cell volume and total plasma protein concentration of blood".
1956 Nicol, B..M, *Brit. J. Nutr.*, 10, 181. "The nutrition of Nigerian children, with reference to their energy requirements".
1956 Nicol, B.M., *Brit. J. Nutr.*, 10, 275. "The nutrition of Nigerian children, with particular reference to their ascorbic acid requirements".
1957 Nicol, B.M., Adviser on Nutrition to the Federal Medical Department, Nigeria, "Standard diet sheets for use in Nigeria". Baraka Press, Kaduna.
1957 Nicol, B.M., *Nature*, 180, 287. "Ascorbic acid content of Baobab fruit".
1958 Nicol, B.M., *West African Med. J.*, 7, 185. "Ascorbic acid in the diets of rural Nigerian people".
1959 Nicol, B.M., *West African Med. J.*, 8, 18. "Fertility and Food in Northern Nigeria".
1959 Nicol, B.M., *Brit. J. Nutr.*, 13, 293. "The Calorie Requirements of Nigerian Peasant Farmers".
1959 Nicol, B.M., *Brit. J. Nutr.*, 13, 307. "The Protein Requirements of Nigerian Peasant Farmers".
1961 Nicol, B.M. and Phillips, P.G., National Academy of Science — National Research Council Publication 843, Washington D.C. "Groundnut Flour and Dried Skimmed Milk as Supplement to the Diets of Nigerian Men and Children".
1963 Nicol, B.M., "The Utilization of Protein-rich Foods in the Prevention of Protein-calorie Deficiency Diseases", Symposia of the Swedish Nutrition Foundation No. 1, p. 152.
1965 Nicol, B.M., "Nutrition in Nigera", prepared for ICNND team, 24461 FAO, Rome.
1965 Nicol, B.M., "Towards Greater Food Supplies", J. Roy Instit. Pub. Health & Hyg., 28, 310.
1967 Nicol, B.M., "Problems concerned with reaching the Pre-school Child". Third Far East Symposium on Nutrition, US National Institutes of Health, Md., p. 114.

LIST OF PUBLICATIONS

1967 Nicol, B.M., "Dietary Bulk as a Factor Influencing Protein and Calorie Intakes", Protein Advisory Group, New York, Document 10/116.
1967/68 Nicol, B.M., "An Indicative Plan for the World". Alfa Laval International, Tumba, Sweden, p. 24.
1970 Nicol, B.M., "Agriculture, Food and Nutrition in Developing Countries", Proceedings of Roy. Soc. Med. *63*, 1177.
1970 Nicol, B.M., "Alias Kwashiorkor", World Review of Animal Production, FAO Special Issue, World Association for Animal Production, Rome, Italy.
1970 Nicol, B.M., "Causes of Famine in the Past and in the Future", Symposia of the Swedish Nutrition Foundation *IX,* p. 10.
1971 Nicol, B.M., "Protein and Calorie Concentration", Nutrition Reviews, *29,* 83.
1971 Nicol, B.M., "Food from Forests", Guinea Zone Conference FAO/IITA, Ibadan, Nigeria, August: FAO, Rome WM/B5854.
1971 Nicol, B.M., "Effect of Climate on Energy and Protein Requirements", FAO, Rome (Ref: ESN:FAO/WHO/PR/71/6e(i)).
1972 Nicol, B.M., "Reasons for, and methods in dietary and food consumption surveys", Proceedings of Symposium of Group of European Nutritionists, Warsaw, April 1972. Bibl. "Nutr. Diet.", No. 20, pp. 69-76: Karger, Basel, 1974.
1973 Nicol, B.M., Consultant report, "Relationship between human food supplies and the prevalence of malnutrition", FAO, Rome.
1973 Nicol, B.M., Consultant report, "Relationship between human food supplies and indicators of health and nutrition", WHO, Geneva.
1974 Nicol, B.M., "Recent developments in the Status of International Food and Nutrition", Proc. Tenth Symp. on Single Cell Protein, Rome, 1973. Academic Press, London (editor, Davis, P.).
1974 Nicol, B.M., "Food and Nutrition in the Agricultural Development Plan for Indonesia". Chapter in report of Food and Planning Team, INS/70/008, FAO, Rome.
1974 Nicol, B.M., "Reasons for, and methods in dietary and food consumption surveys", (Warsaw) Nutr. Diet No. 20, pp. 69-76, Karger, Basel.

LIST OF PUBLICATIONS

1974 Passmore, R., Nicol, B.M. and M. Narayana Rao (1974), "Handbook on Human Nutritional Requirements", WHO, Geneva, WHO Monograph Series, No. 61.

1975 Nicol, B.M., "Food and Nutrition in Malaysia's Development Planning". Consultant report, Ref. No. RAFE 20, FAO, Bangkok.

1976 Nicol, B.M., "Endogenous nitrogen extraction and utilization of dietary protein", *Brit. J. Nutr.* (1976), *35*, 181.

1976 Nicol, B.M. and Phillips, P.G., "The utilization of dietary protein by Nigerian men", *Brit. J. Nutr.*, *36*, 337.

1978 Nicol, B.M. and Phillips, P.G., "The utilization of proteins and amino acids in diets based on cassava (*Manihot utilissima*), rice or sorghum (*Sorghum sativa*) by young Nigerian men of low income", *Brit. J. Nutr.* (1978) *39*, 271.

1980 Nicol, B.M., "Sickling among Todas in Nilgiris, S. Indian: 'Daddawa' as food in Nigeria". *Ecology Food and Nutr.*, *10*, 61.

Other Communications and Addresses

1938 To Gastro-Enterological Club at Cambridge: "Standard diet Sheets for use in Nigeria", Baraka Press Ltd., Kaduna, Nigeria.

1961 Address to American Food for Peace Council, First Regional Conference, Great Plains Region, Denver, November 20.

1962 Report to Committee on Protein Malnutrition of the US Food and Nutrition Board — Possibilities for Implementation of the Committee's Protein-Rich Food Research Programme in Latin America.

1967 Report to 43rd Session of UN Economic and Social Council, Geneva, July on "Increasing the Production and Use of Edible Protein".

1971 Note on Protein/Nitrogen/Amino acid requirements of adult Nigerian men for maintenance, to Protein Requirements Committee, FAO/WHO.

1971 Notes for talk to NUFFIC Course on Uist, 12/13 July.

1971 "Climate", FAO/WHO Ad Hoc Committee of Experts on Energy and Proteins, Requirements and Recommended Intakes. ESN: FAO/WHO/PR/71/6e(i) — FAO WM/B 2408.

1972 "Nutritional Improvement of Food Legumes by Breeding", PAG Symposium, Rome, p. 53.
1972 January, Statement to WHO Executive Board.
1972 Talk to Planning for Better Family Living Orientation Seminar (Home Economics), July 1971.

List of Illustrations

Dr Bruce Nicol	Frontispiece
Territorial Royal Signals, the author on left.	46
Brigadier Glyn Hughes on right, talking to Her Majesty Queen Elizabeth at Guards Armoured Division HQ, Wincanton, prior to landing at Normandy on D-Day plus 1. The author is behind Queen Elizabeth's hat.	46
Preparation of gari from peeled cassava root, Ughelli, August 1949.	119
Christmas Eve 1952, in a canoe near the source of the River Niger in Nigeria.	122
The author with staff of Kaduna Hospital and Christopher.	124
With nutrition unit, Kaduna.	128
Diana with straw canoe near Lake Chad.	140
A catch of Lake Chad fish (large ones are Heterotis).	141
The author's wife and daughter.	145
Drum when beaten summons workers in the fields.	147
En route to market, five miles north of Yelwa.	149

Foreword

In his working life Bruce Nicol made valuable contributions to our knowledge of nutrition in general and in particular to the problems in the Third World. His close association with these in Nigeria gave him an unrivalled understanding of the social and other causes of malnutrition in poor countries and he made very effective use of this knowledge in the planning and development of the nutrition programmes of the UN agencies in the poorer countries throughout the world.

Dr J. BURGESS

OBITUARY

Dr Bruce Nicol

The death of Dr. Bruce Nicol in England has deprived *Ecology of Food and Nutrition* of one of its most valuable counsellors and reviewers. Dr. Nicol was involved in the genesis of the journal and throughout the eighteen years of his membership of the Editorial Board he gave contributors and readers the benefit of his fine brain, his exacting critical review skills, and his profound knowledge of nutritional problems in the Third World.

Bruce Milligan Nicol was born in Ayrshire, Scotland, in 1913, the first son of a Minister of the Church of Assembly of Scotland. His primary and secondary school education was at Edinburgh Academy where he excelled at learning, cricket, and rugby football. Although medicine was not his first choice as a career, he abandoned banking as an alternative after the premature death of his father. Recognising that his mother would be preoccupied with the raising of her five other children he was encouraged to enter Medical School by his maternal grandmother. His intellectual prowess enabled him to win several scholarships which helped to overcome the financial problems of his widowed mother. He qualified as a physician from Aberdeen University in 1935. In his immediate postgraduate career he worked for Professors Learmonth and Stanley Davidson. When the latter, an outstanding figure in medical science, moved to Edinburgh University, Nicol followed. In this stimulating environment, Nicol's interests matured, and focused on peptic ulcer disease. His clinical work and research were supplemented by a stint as a ship's surgeon. In this vocation he obtained a wider exposure to medicine and his knowledge of ulcers was augmented by visits to hospitals in his ports of call in India and the Far East. He was settling down to a career as an 'ulcer specialist' and had published his first paper on the subject in the *Lancet* in 1939.

OBITUARY

Prior to this, however, in 1933, he had joined the famous 51st Highland Division as a Territorial Officer in the Royal Army Signal Corps. He was sent to France in a non-medical role at the outbreak of hostilities. His qualifications in medicine did not go unnoticed and he was transferred to the Royal Army Medical Corps. This was indeed fortunate as his original unit was captured when France fell to the Germans, with the result that his mother was erroneously notified that he was 'missing, believed killed'.

While other units of the British Army were evacuating from Dunkirk, Nicol was in hiding near Cherbourg. He eventually escaped by boat and landed back in England at Poole in Dorset. (A location close to where he made his home in retirement for many years.) After an assignment with Combined Operations which presented Britain with the only opportunity for offensive operations in Europe at that time, he transferred to the Guards Armoured Division. In this unit, in command of the 19th Light Field Ambulance, he went back to France on D-Day. He was awarded the Order of the British Empire (OBE Military Division) for his work at the Battle of Arnhem. He was the youngest lieutenant-colonel in the Guards Armoured Division, he still had not received a commission in the Royal Army Medical Corps so he transferred to the Colonial Medical Service and was assigned to Nigeria.

As a District Medical Officer in Northern Nigeria he became interested in what Nigerians were eating, and their reasons for choosing that particular food. Unlike so many expatriates, he recognised that the European diet was not the standard by which all diets should be judged, and he diligently started documenting food intakes and exploring the nutritional value of local foods. After his first tour of duty he was transferred to the Bight of Benin where his interest in nutritional science grew. He persuaded the government to establish a Nutrition Unit and as the Federal Nutrition Adviser, and with the assistance of Peter Phillips, his laboratory assistant, his research on diet, growth, and seasonal food patterns became more productive and he published extensively in the leading journals. The topics included 'Tribal Nutrition and Health', 'Beta lipoprotein and cholesterol concentrations in Nigeria' as well as evaluations of methodologists used for the assessment of nutritional status, and the use of protein supplements as a means of preventing malnutrition. His influence

OBITUARY

became international and he made significant contributions to the London University/FAO/WHO International Nutrition Seminar in Kampala in 1958. Further publications at this time focused on problems of dietary and food consumption surveys, famine, indigenous foods with special reference to the potential role of forest foods, and protein requirements.

After Nigeria achieved political independence from Britain, Nicol joined FAO. His first assignment was as a Liaison Officer with UNICEF in New York. UNICEF staff still recognise the tremendous contributions he made to achieving an understanding of the Alfatoxin problem in tropically grown ground (pea) nuts and its role in the genesis of liver cancer. It will be recalled that this was a staggering problem at that time as ground nut production was thought to be vital to Third World countries.

In 1962 he was assigned to FAO headquarters in Rome as Deputy Director of the Nutritions Division (and later as Acting Director during the prolonged illness of Marcel Autret). In these positions he continued to guide FAO policies on Nutrition in the Third World by organising conferences, and through FAO publications. Like so many of us who served with FAO and WHO at that time he became frustrated with the interminable disputes over demarcation of the respective responsibilities of the two agencies, and the policies that negated much of their effective function. The result was his early retirement.

This was fortunate for *Ecology of Food and Nutrition* for he was able to devote much time and energy to the solution of the problems which arose during the journal's gestation. His work had demonstrated to him, without doubt, that food and health could not be separated into two distinct branches of science. He was also aware of the role of human behaviour as a determinant of nutritional status and health. This concept was unusual thirty years ago, and it is largely due to Nicol's support that the Editorial Board was able to implement a policy that brought behavioural sciences such as anthropology and sociology (and associated sciences such as archaeology and ethnobotany) into the nutritional arena. He also supported our belief that there was a vast amount of publishable scientifically sound research being carried out in remote areas of the world. He urged that researchers be encouraged to write up their results and let them pass the scrutiny of critical reviewers in the Western Hemisphere.

OBITUARY

During his service to the journal, Nicol became one of its most important reviewers. He had unlimited patience and he would spend considerable amounts of time (and much of his own money) cajoling contributors to try harder. He was highly critical of scientific content and grammar, and woe betide any potential author who tried to introduce modern clichés, or jargon, into the text in order to be fashionable. A review of the content and character of the journal from its inception demonstrates his strong and lasting influence. The journal is international and eclectic and this latter characteristic, as well as its high standards, are a direct result of his efforts. What is not apparent is his devotion to this work. Crippled by a stroke, and subsequent injuries resulting from this affliction, he continued to be helpful and productive, and he was undoubtedly the backbone of our review process to the end. He is sorely missed as a colleague and although we only met four times over a period of thirty-five years he will also be missed as a personal friend. To his wife Mary, who also has given unstinted help to the journal by helping with typing and other burdensome chores, and his family, we extend our deepest sympathy.

Dr J. K. Robson, MD, Editor
Ecology of Food and Nutrition
Volume 24

CHAPTER 1

Family Background

The manse of Skelmorlie, where I was born on 24 March 1913, looks over the Firth of Clyde with beautiful views of the Isle of Bute, the Cumbrae Islands and, on fine days, the island of Arran. My father, David Bruce Nicol, was minister of the parish from July 1911 to May 1916 and then from July 1919 to September 1920. My earliest memories of life there include learning how to light a bonfire under instruction from the gardener and having my own dog, a golden-brown labrador. Milk was delivered from dairy to door in a model-T Ford and I recollect going around in the van, driven by a milkmaid, not a milkman, during wartime.

Immediately below the manse, on the Firth of Clyde, ships built in the busy Clyde and Glasgow yards carried out their trials along the official 'measured mile' and I remember seeing the battleship HMS *Hood* there before the end of the war. Airships used that stretch of river to carry out their trials, too. When the Clyde Regatta was restarted after the war we saw J class yachts, such as *Britannia*, *Astra* and *Endeavour* competing across the estuary.

I had a governess who tutored me until I took the entrance examination for Edinburgh Academy under her supervision, at home, in the spring of 1920.

My father was an Edinburgh man; he was born in the city in 1886. My grandfather was Professor of Biblical Criticism at Aberdeen University and it was at that university that father, too, was educated, graduating as a Bachelor of Divinity in 1908. He had also read medicine for one year but decided that his real vocation lay in the Church. He was ordained as minister of the Church of Scotland at Skelmorlie in 1911 and married in April the following year.

As soon as war broke out my father wanted to join up, but as a chaplain, not as a fighting man. He was unable to obtain his commission until 1916. Thereafter he served in France, Macedonia and Thessalonia and Palestine. In April 1918, still chaplain, my father was transferred to France with his division. After the fighting around Henin Hill, north of Arras, he was awarded the Military Cross for 'attending to the wounded with utter disregard for danger, under intense fire'. About this time he was also mentioned in dispatches.

After the Armistice he found it as difficult to get out of the army as it had been to get in to it. He stayed with his battalion in Belgium until spring 1919, then with the 1st Battalion Black Watch in Aldershot, where he was attached to St Andrew's Church of Scotland. He was Presbyterian Chaplain of the Royal Military College at Sandhurst. Eventually, by mid-July 1919, he was demobilised and back in Skelmorlie.

Life in his country parish made him restless after his experiences of war and he gladly took the opportunity that was offered to him of moving the family to Edinburgh and taking the parish of St Margaret's, with the practical training of divinity students at the university under his charge. The possibility of working in a slum area appealed to him greatly and he was pleased, too, at the facilities which existed for our future education. I was by now the eldest of three: my sister Betty, (Elizabeth Ann Underwood) was two years younger, and Tom (Thomas James Trail) was nearly four years my junior.

Owing to the interest in genealogy shown by several members of my family and, in particular, by my father and grandfather Trail and a cousin, Colonel Claud Moir, I have been able to gain much information about my family's history. Several of my Nicol kinsmen did well for themselves in business, became landowners or worked in the academic and professional fields.

In 1879 my grandfather Nicol became minister of the ancient Tolbooth Parish Church, in the Royal Mile, Edinburgh. He remained there until gaining the Chair of Divinity and Biblical Criticism in Aberdeen University in 1899, an appointment he held until his death in 1916. He was Moderator of the General Assembly of the Church of Scotland in 1914.

My mother, Helen Trail, was born at 81 High Street, Old Aberdeen, in 1887, Queen Victoria's Golden Jubilee year. She went to school first at the Misses Bowmans' school for young children of the Old Town, boys and girls. When fifteen she was sent to the Ministers' Daughters' College in Edinburgh, 'principally I think because your father and I were supposed to be seeing too much of one another'. She left the MDC when she was eighteen and was sent to Hanover to be 'finished' and to learn German. 'But, alas, I got in tow with a lot of English boys who were being tutored for Sandhurst and most of my time was spent playing hockey and tennis with them. I had a delightful room on the ground floor with a balcony overlooking Arneswaldstrasse. I enjoyed myself extremely and learnt no German.'

The family (my father and mother, my sister Betty, aged five, brother Tom aged three and myself aged seven) moved to Edinburgh in September 1920. The parish of St Margaret's Church, Dumbiedykes, my father's new charge, consisted mainly of tenements at the lower end of Arthur Street, not far from the Palace of Holyroodhouse. A manse was not provided with the church, and eventually my parents settled for a Georgian house of three storeys and a basement in the New Town in Saxe Coburg Place, which was only a short walk from Edinburgh Academy where I was to start school in October. A few days after we had settled into number 31 Saxe Coburg Place, my mother, paying no heed to my perturbation, took me into the gardens to meet some boys who were playing 'touch rugger' and to introduce herself, and me, to them. The eldest of the boys, who was then twelve years of age, introduced himself as Ronnie Wright, of number 12, and his younger brother Selby, and Phil Wood and Bob Wood of number 15. Mother explained I was going to start my first term at the Academy at the beginning of October and was rather nervous about it. Ronnie immediately assured me that 'we are all Academy boys here; we will keep an eye on you'. Which they all did, very kindly, and Bob Wood, about nine months my senior, became one of only two *very* good friends I made at the Academy although I had many others made in the ordinary course of school activities.

The Woods played a large part in my life, while I was at the Academy and afterwards, but the Wrights left school in 1924 to go to Melville College and I lost touch with them. My brother Tom has worked with Ronnie during the course of their army careers and in other aspects of the work of the Church of Scotland.

At school, as well as passing the Oxford and Cambridge School Certificate and the Scottish Higher School Leaving Certificate I developed a love for cricket, rugby football, rugby fives, military rifle shooting and of Gilbert and Sullivan operas and the possibility of singing and acting in them; and a grounding in the nature of the army through the Officers' Training Corps. All this indicates the nature and quality of the Edinburgh Academy, which, I am glad to say, has improved and widened since my days there. My nine years at the Academy fell into three different periods depending on my family's residential status. From October 1920 to December 1925 I was a day boy living at home in 31 Saxe Coburg Place. At the beginning of the Easter term of 1926, when my father was given charge of St Mark's Church in Dundee, I boarded at 15 Saxe Coburg Place, with the parents of Phil and Bob Wood — the Major, a Yorkshireman, was posted to the Military Hospital, Edinburgh Castle, as pathologist. I lived with the Woods until he retired and they moved to their house in Peeblesshire, Scotston, in 1928. My last year at the Academy was as a boarder in Scott House.

In my day the great preponderance of Academy masters were English with excellent academic backgrounds from Oxford and Cambridge. The greatest emphasis in the teaching from the beginning was classical but the natural sciences had crept in before I went to school, and were greatly expanded during my time there. With the overall emphasis on classics, the curriculum covered history, geography, French or German. Latin was obligatory for all, including those going up the science side, as I did.

I cannot remember that I ever felt overworked or worried about my academic studies, a good mark for the quality of our form masters. It seemed more important to get one's 'colours' at cricket or rugger. I achieved this ambition at cricket but not at rugger. I was disappointed to be dropped from the shooting eight to the Cadet Fair for Bisley, but it was the year (1928) that the eight won the Country Life Trophy (first at 500 yards in the Ashburton Shield competition).

During my spell at the Academy (1920-1929) there were two Rectors (headmasters), R. H. Ferard, MA(Oxon), LLD(Edin), and Mr P. H. B. Lyon, MD, MA(Oxon), who was appointed headmaster of Rugby in 1931. Dr. Ferard we found 'very boring', his short addresses at morning prayers being, we thought, 'dull'.

Mr Lyon, on the other hand, having been in the Great War, was much more interesting and entertaining to us. In 1932, when I required referees' reports to support my application for a commission in the Territorial Army, I received the following note from him from the School House, Rugby:

3rd March 1932
My Dear Nicol,
I have signed the enclosed forms and return them herewith. I have rashly testified to your character for the past six years, so I hope you haven't gone irretrievably to the bad since I last saw you.
Yours very sincerely,
P. Hugh B. Lyon.

For many of the masters, too many to mention individually, I had a great respect and liking. Mr E. R. Hempson MA(Cantab), FRGS, not only taught English and geography imaginatively, but also appeared in the 'Free and Easy' (the school concert at the end of term at Easter) in comical songs with the bald-headed 'Pa-Mo' (Mr J. L. Mosley, MA(Oxon)). Mr Hempson had a good tenor voice and acted in the annual Gilbert and Sullivan operettas which were produced towards the end of each summer term from 1922 until 1928. He was a notable Nanki Poo to my classmate, Tae Tod's Yum Yum in *The Mikado* (1923). I reached the dizzy heights of being understudy to Pish Tush in that production.

I must not omit Mr B. G. W. Atkinson, MA(Cantab), who was in charge of cricket and was house tutor at Jeffrey House. He played for Middlesex during the summer holidays, and it was he who, by raising his bat over his head with both arms, smashed a bouncer from A. R. Gover of Surrey for a straight six into the Lords Pavilion.

It would be remiss of me, when speaking of the Academy, to omit reference to our sports field, Raeburn Place, a ground of much character (particularly before 'The Mound' was levelled) and of great historic interest to present-day Rugby Union football fans. Rugger was first played in Scotland at Raeburn Place. It was here that the first international match took place between Scotland and England in 1871 and here most of Scotland's home matches were played until 1899.

While the family lived at 31 Saxe Coburg Place my father had many interesting visitors, some of whom we children were allowed to meet. Many were ex-army friends who came only for a gossip about war experiences, but some were ex-officers or other ranks who could not find work in the slump of the early 1920s, and were asking for help. Others were professional colleagues, ministers of the Church of Scotland or priests of other denominations, Roman Catholics, Anglicans and the Episcopalian Church of Scotland.

Apart from the blight of Miss F., who had little to do with me as I was at school, but made Betty and Tom miserable from time to time, 31 Saxe Coburg Place was a happy house. I was given a Raleigh bicycle and Bob Wood and I learned to cycle around Saxe Coburg Place. We had a small garden behind with a greenhouse in which I kept tortoises, a very large larder off the kitchen, which I raided regularly for raisins and currants with the connivance of Annie, the cook who came from the Duke of Atholl's estate at Blair Castle, Perthshire. Father had befriended her when she had some social trouble at home and she was our cook for many years, in Skelmorlie, Edinburgh and in Dundee.

The Christmas gift of a 'pogo stick', upon which we became experts in the ground-floor day nursery, was an expensive error on the part of my parents. When I was jumping well on it one day I was surprised to find myself suspended by my arms, one on each side of a hole in the floor through which my vehicle had vanished into the maid's bedroom in the basement below. This was the way the dry rot, which pervaded the ground floor room, was diagnosed. It caused a lot of inconvenience and expense to have the floors relaid but the price of the house must have been increased when it was sold. 'Thirty-one' was the location of my first introduction to obstetrics. I kept, quite licitly, in a cardboard box under my bed, a pair of white mice. I was nearly sick one morning when, on going to give the mice their day's rations, I found a horrible wriggling mass of small pink things which had not been there the night before. This may have been a factor leading to my preference for medicine and surgery over obstetrics and gynaecology. The incident gave my mother a great deal of amusement and a good opportunity to introduce me to some of the basic facts of life.

FAMILY BACKGROUND

Going to church on Sunday mornings, I was amazed by the number of men sleeping on the pavements or in the gutters. It was explained that they were ex-servicemen who could not get work or find anywhere to stay on account of something called 'the slump', which was never defined in a way I could understand at seven or eight years of age. A decade later as a medical student assisting in the casualty department of the Aberdeen Royal Infirmary on Saturday nights or Sunday mornings the next 'slump' taught me to what lengths people accustomed to work, who find themselves unemployed, will go to escape for a few hours the current realities of life. Apart from attempted suicide (drinking carbolic acid was then a popular method), a mixture of cheap red wine and methylated spirits, Brasso or Silvo strained through a cloth, or even drunk neat, taught one how to use the stomach pump, but irreversible damage was often done before attention could be given to those unfortunates. In the present (1986) wave of unemployment many of the 3.5 million non-workers have never worked at all since leaving school, probably did not work much while at school, have not experienced discipline in a satisfactory form either in the home or at school, and one gets the impression the Welfare State and successive governments have let them down. Such present-day unemployed do not seem inclined to want to work and stand on their own feet. They, especially the young, pass their time in much more sinister ways than those in vogue in the early 1920s and early 1930s, embracing as they do petty or major crime, 'mugging', hard drugs, sexual licence and perversion and often become unfortunately, crypto-communists. Such is the effect, I fear, of Beveridge's Plan and the Welfare State in a so-called democratic and free country. 'None can love freedom heartily, but good men; the rest love not freedom, but licence' (Milton).

In her eighty-ninth year, my mother noted: 'Now universities are crowded out by students whose fees are paid by government grants, they have long hair, run their own cars on their grants, get married (some of them) and get an extra £500 a year — and this is *not* as it should be. It is very sad and of the permissive society I most thoroughly disapprove. I'm only too glad that it was given to me to bring up the six of you when what I said had to be done, and when young people didn't get their pockets full of money as they do now.' This anticipates the births of my sister Margaret Helen Scott (always known as Susan or Sue) in Edinburgh in 1924, David Mark Wotherspoon (Mark) in Dundee in 1926, and Kenneth Moir (Ken) also in Dundee in 1928. '*Your* families have all been well brought up, I'm glad to say, and I have sixteen delightful grandchildren.'

Each year the family went on holiday to a large farm called Pittarig, near Moulin on the road from Pitlochry via Kirkmichael to Blairgowrie. Here I started my hill walking and mountaineering experiences on Ben Vrackie, and short-distance bicycle tours with my father. We would set out early in the morning and ride to the Queen's View on Loch Tummel and look at the cone of Schiehallion in the west, a mountain I have never climbed; or we would go through the Pass of Killiecrankie past Blair Castle and take the path to the Falls of Bruar, whence looking north one saw the hills of the Forest of Atholl. As we got older such bicycling expeditions increased in length and scope and included Betty and eventually Tom by 1924. We helped the farmer harvesting the oats (known as 'corn' on the highlands of Scotland) and my first earned money (half a crown) was paid to me by him for 'lifting' storm-flattened corn ahead of the reaper, long before the combine harvester was known. We tied the corn into bundles and built them into 'stooks', each stook being six bundles.

When the family moved to Dundee in 1925, we lived in No. 9 Airlie Place, a street which included several doctors and other professional and businessmen among its residents.

I kept diaries covering most of my school holidays, illustrated by snapshots taken with small and primitive cameras, and recorded the various cycling and fishing trips undertaken with Bob Wood usually in the Borders. We were also starting to be keen ornithologists from 1925 onwards.

At the beginning of the 1927 session a boy came to the Academy who became one of my best friends. His name was Patrick Baird, of whom I saw a lot both at school and afterwards. One does not choose friends. One drifts into friendships which revive quickly even after long absences. It was so with myself and Pat Baird and with Bob Wood. After the long period of my absence from the United Kingdom during the Second World War, in Africa and in Italy, lasting from 1939 to 1977, I seldom heard from or of either of them until Pat wrote from Canada about 1980 and proposed himself for a visit to us in our house in Dorset. His visit was delightful and as satisfying a way of bridging the long gap in our contacts as one could have wished.

The story of my schooldays finishes with the 1929 Exhibition at school and the OTC camp at Elie in Fife. That camp was a very successful one for the Academy. We won all the competitions; including the pipe band and individual piping events, and, most important of all, the Guard Competition. Being slightly over six feet at that time I was the right marker for fixing bayonets, had the ordeal of taking those six paces forwards! As I recollect Pat Baird, also tall, was the left marker. However, all went well and we celebrated our victory heartily in the canteen on lemonade shandy and pork pies. Then back to school after our 0200 reveille to hand in our OTC kit and arms and make our various ways into the great world beyond the shelter of school.

CHAPTER 2

Youth and Medical Studies

At the end of my schooldays I had not the remotest idea what work I wanted to do. I had good university entrance qualifications, but no desire to take up any particular profession. Therefore my father had made arrangements through a wartime friend who, in 1929, was a senior official in the Union Bank of Scotland Ltd., in London, that I start a five-year apprenticeship to that bank in Glasgow. My father had already been selected to take charge of Govan Old Parish Church, a famous old pre-Reformation institution — now Established Church of Scotland.

I went to the bank in Bothwell Street from Monday to Friday by bus at 8 a.m., leaving when the day's balance had been struck. Very occasionally my father and mother would come into central Glasgow to give me dinner and then go on to a theatre. A group of admirable players were by good fortune having one of their last seasons in Scotland in the winter of 1929. I had seen them before in London once or twice. This group were the Co-optimists which included amongst its members Melville Gideon, Laddie Cliff, Ivy St. Helier, Elsa Macfarlane, Phyllis Monkman, who sang 'The Rolls Royce Lady', Clifford Gray, Davy Burnaby, and Stanley Holloway. They were particular favourites of my father's and how competent and cheerful they were! Few people now remember them, but I still have some of their sheet music inherited from my father.

In early March 1930 I was not feeling very well and our new general practitioner found some 'albumin' in my urine and confined me to bed with a diagnosis of acute nephritis, although I did not pass any blood, did not have any fever, and with hindsight was probably only suffering from adolescent albuminaria. My young sister Susan definitely had an acute nephritis from which she recovered rapidly. Father was taken seriously ill with what

YOUTH AND MEDICAL STUDIES

was, I believe correctly, diagnosed as acute streptococcal nephritis. My Aunt Dorothy came through from her wards in the Edinburgh Royal Infirmary, where she was a Sister, to help with the nursing, but after three weeks he relapsed into a coma and died on 23 March 1930, the day before my seventeenth birthday, at the age of forty-four years.

This tragedy was difficult to comprehend for several days, and it was not until after the funeral in Govan Parish Church and his burial in the St Machar's Cathedral churchyard, Old Aberdeen, that mother started to wonder what was to be done.

In 1933 a memorial to my father was unveiled in the Steven Chapel of Govan Parish Church by my grand-uncle, the Very Reverend Professor George Milligan. The memorial was erected by his many friends and takes the form of a carved oak reredos screen placed above the altar and under the chapel's cross, illuminated by a bronze lamp suspended from the ceiling.

It was decided by my mother and Trail grandmother that the best thing to do, in the first instance, was to move the family to 81 High Street, Old Aberdeen, the large house which my grandfather Trail had purchased in 1879 when he became Professor of Botany in Aberdeen University. There was ample room for our whole family, my grandmother and Aunt Brenda (Auntie Tam, my mother's youngest sister). The question of my embryonic banking career was left to me to fix with my father's friend in London, the one who had arranged for me to join the bank. I had already decided that such an occupation was not for me, and that I would like to study medicine. Why this idea came to me I still do not know though there were several precedents in the family. If it had any relationship with my father's untimely death, it must have been an unconscious reaction, and I really do not believe in that kind of psychology. I consider it one of the winds of chance which have blown through my life at moments of crisis or importance.

My mother felt that I should stick to the original contract I had signed with the bank at five years duration but my grandmother produced one of the compromises for which her life had so well fitted her to make. She was desperately keen that I should read medicine at Aberdeen, but did not want to upset my mother at the start of her long period of bringing up a family without the aid of a husband. Thus my grandmother proposed that I should approach the bank asking for a transfer to an Aberdeen branch in the immediate future, and at the same time I study for a Carnegie scholarship, being tutored by the reader in zoology, who worked in that department of which Sir Arthur Thomas was professor. I was to tell the bank of this proposal, and ask for its permission to leave the bank if I was successful. To this approach my father's friend in London agreed. I was duly posted to the Fishmarket branch of the Union Bank in Aberdeen. As my physics and chemistry from school were adequate, I had to concentrate on zoology and botany for the scholarship, which I eventually obtained in July of 1930. It is of interest that Mr Neill, who tutored me, lived in the same house in the High Street, Old Aberdeen, which had been the school run by the Misses Bowman, where my mother first went to school and where I studied for the scholarship which provided more than half of the university fees and books for the five-year course. I received a small allowance from my mother and my grandmother paid the balance of the university fees.

I started my medical studies in October 1930, while the family was still living in 81 High Street. My grandmother had agreed, very generously, to build a house for us on a site which was available in Springfield Road, a new road being developed in what was then country on the western outskirts of Aberdeen. The house was ready for occupation in 1931. My mother had a small widow's pension from the Church of Scotland and a private income which was not inconsiderable so that the family could live quite comfortably in number 222 Springfield Road when it was completed.

I lived at '222', as the house became known throughout the family, during the whole five years of the medical course. My sisters Betty and Susan went to St Leonard's School at St Andrews, Fife, where my grandmother Trail/Milligan had been a former pupil. My younger brother Tom went to the Aberdeen Grammar School, having had one year at the Edinburgh Academy (1924-25) before we moved to Dundee, where he attended the Dundee High School, and then to Glasgow Academy for a few months during our short and tragic stay in Glasgow. Younger brothers Mark and Kenneth, when they reached school age, were educated at the Aberdeen Grammar School.

Learning to Practise the Art of Medicine: Pre-clinical Days
    I was very fortunate in starting my medical studies at Aberdeen in 1930 as the numbers of medical students at that time were

not as excessive as they became within five years. My class of 1930-35 numbered fifty in all, eight were female and forty-two male students. This section of my book is for the information of my family and non-medical friends.

Medicine, with a capital M, depends largely on the natural sciences of chemistry (inorganic and organic), botany, zoology, physiology and anatomy. At Aberdeen University in the 1930s study of these sciences was undertaken in the first two years of the curriculum.

I needed to learn as much as I could of what was then known of the relationship between organic chemistry and physiology and as I recollect this aspect of the subject was taught very well. Professor Craib, who had taken over the Botany Department from my grandfather Trail in 1920, tried to teach 'botany' rather than the qualities of plants as remedial agents for use in medical practice, a subject which, I have been told, was one of my grandfather's *tours de force*. Professor Alexander (Daddy) Lowe gave an excellent systematic course of lectures in anatomy, and kept very accurate data on certain aspects of the skeletal sizes of all his students, male and female, which he had been compiling over three decades. These data demonstrated the increasing stature of young men and women in the age group seventeen to twenty-two years during the period from the turn of the century to 1931. In 1930 I had the doubtful distinction of having the longest spine in relation to my total height of all the data recorded by that year. This means that my legs (and arms) are relatively short, and this is a generic characteristic shared by me with my brothers and sisters, and my own son and daughter. I inherited the trait from my father, although we were both six feet two inches (1.88m) at the age of forty years.

Most of our practical anatomical knowledge was derived from dissection of the human body in the 'drain', the large and airy room in the Anatomy Department where the corpses were laid out on their individual slate tables. The two 'demonstrators' on the Anatomy Department staff, one of whom was Norman Logie, who became a very competent surgeon and good friend of mine, were very important in organising one's methods of dissection of whatever 'part' (head and neck, thorax, lower extremity, etc.) of the body on which one was working at any given time. The lecturer in anatomy, Dr Robert Lockhart, was doing research on the mobility of muscles and of joints, using a trained young female ballet dancer as a model. Unfortunately we only saw the X-ray pictures which he took of this girl! The obituary of Professor Lockhart, who succeeded Professor Lowe and remained in that chair for thirty-two years, was published in the *Daily Telegraph* of 4 March 1987. He had reached the age of ninety-three years.

My copy of Grey's *Anatomy*, the standard textbook of the time, was inherited from my grandfather's library; its date was 1915! Only two years ago I was shown, by a physiotherapist who was helping me recover the use of my left limbs following a cerebral embolism, the most recent edition dated 1984 and, apart from some minor changes in terminology, the most noticeable advance made in the science of anatomy seemed to me to be the increased knowledge of joint capsules and the potential movement of joints in people who are physically well trained.

Botany and zoology, chemistry and physics were completed in the first year of the five-year course, but anatomy, physiology and biochemistry were spread over the first two years. The science of physiology, including biochemistry which was taught to us as a separate subject in the Physiology Department, is, to the embryo medical practitioner, by far the most important aspect of the 'premedical' curriculum.

We were fortunate in having Professor J. J. M. Macleod, FRS, as head of the Physiology Department. He had only recently returned to Aberdeen from being Professor of Physiology at McGill University, Toronto. It was under his overall direction in that Canadian department that Banting and Best had discovered insulin, and assessed the action of the hormone in the human species. One could say that this was a 'rediscovery' of insulin, as a substance with insulin-like properties and activity had been isolated from fish pancreas just before the 1914-18 war in the Zoology Department of Aberdeen University by Dr Kelly. This work was never properly followed up. We were also fortunate in having Dr Cleghorn, a Canadian biochemist/physiologist in the department, and I think it was from him that I learned most of the physiology I knew when we sat the pre-clinical examination in this subject.

At the end of the second year all the pre-clinical work was finished and examinations passed without too many qualms.

YOUTH AND MEDICAL STUDIES

Holidays between Terms and Sessions

The close friends I made during the first year of our course, and with whom I kept in touch for many years, were Alec Keith (nephew of Sir Arthur Keith, the anthropologist) from Fettes, Peter Ingram from Westminster, Montie Maconachy from Merchiston, Phillip Mitchell, son of Dr. Mitchell of Old Aberdeen, who lived opposite 81 High Street and had been at the Edinburgh Academy with me, Alexander Slessor (Sandy) from Inverness, and Stewart Slessor from Frazerburgh. I had a good companion keen on climbing, from Robert Gordon's College, Aberdeen, Ian Duthie. Phillip Mitchell's elder brother, Stephen, who was three years older than Phillip, had always been stage-struck and played a realistic Dick Dead Eye in *HMS Pinafore* and the Judge in *Trial by Jury* when they were put on at school in 1922 and 1923. He became an impresario in London, sponsoring many successful London West end productions.

From 1932 to 1935 four of us, Alec Keith, Monty Maconachy, Stewart Slessor and I spent two weeks of each Easter vacation climbing and ski-ing in the Cairngorms. We based ourselves at Maggie Gruar's cottage in Inverey, six miles west of Braemar near the Linn of Dee on the south bank. We had four beds in a well-built wooden hut behind her cottage. She gave us bacon, egg and sausage for breakfast at 7 a.m. sharp, and we did the rest of our catering ourselves on primus stoves. We learned a lot about the beautiful Cairngorms, usually deep in snow in April. We had to carry our skis or climb on skins if we felt like it. The downhill runs we got were well worth the effort. We enjoyed dining in the Fife Arms in Braemar in the evenings.

Social Life during my Medical Course

I made many other friends on the rugby field and playing cricket. The university had a number of Jamaican medical students either ahead of or behind my year, but we all played cricket, especially one by the name of A. A. Peat and another called Glen Campbell, who were high-class performers. I was to meet them again years later in their own country. During my first year I cannot remember that I was at all interested in girls, being content to relax with the rugger or cricket team on Saturday evenings over more or less beer in the medical students' favourite hostelries. On occasions we would bail out a friend who had

15

committed some small indiscretion from the cells, the fee being set always at ten shillings.

After living in Aberdeen for a year and at the beginning of my second academic session I became aware of the fact that certain girls were considerably more interesting than others. This did not only relate to good looks but also to that indefinable something which used to be called 'sex appeal' or the power of attracting the opposite sex. I began to realise that 'a woman is a dish for the gods, if the devil dress her not' (Shakespeare). Unfortunately, owing to the taboos which applied in my family and in the families of most of my friends and of my girlfriends, sex appeal might incite desire, often mutual, but pre-marital relationships were, in those days, out of the question due our strict education in morals and manners. Hence such friendships were seldom long lasting, but became more and more frequent.

My girlfriends fell into two main categories, due to my position as an undergraduate and my family background. The first group were university students, budding medical practitioners, mostly in academic years junior to mine. Others were daughters of friends of my family who lived in Aberdeen. Such girls, mostly younger, but some older than me, were readily available and more or less willing to be taken to dances, or 'hops' as we used to call them, on Saturday nights at the University Union in Marischal College or in the Palais-de-danse in Union Street.

Then there were the girls whose parents had estates in Aberdeenshire and Kincardine. Many of these families seemed to have a superfluity of girls, such as my cousins the Pauls of Dainston, on the Don, who had three girls (Mary, Dorothy and Enid) but no sons. Many of these families gave 'balls' during the Deeside autumn season and eligible young men were at a premium to act as partners for their daughters. I received many invitations from kind parents. Having a car was a bonus as I could help to ferry my partner and others from house to house, sometimes being asked to stay with one or other set of parents, more often having to drive myself back to Aberdeen in the later hours of the early morning, i.e. before breakfast. The main event of the season was the Aboyne Ball, held towards the end of August. It was customary to make up parties of four or eight of us for this ball so that we could practice beforehand for the reels which formed a large number of the dances on one's programme. The other dances

YOUTH AND MEDICAL STUDIES

such as old-fashioned waltzes and foxtrots were carefully allocated to us by friends.

I started going to these Aberdeenshire parties when a third-year medical student in 1933 and continued on and off until I was an assistant in the Department of Medicine at Aberdeen University, in 1937 and 1938. On one occasion, when I was staying at 81 High Street with my grandmother, she said: 'You got home at half-past five this morning. Where did you come back from? I saw from your white tie you must have been to a ball.' I replied, saying that I had been to a dance at the Vaughan-Lees' house near Kincardine O'Neil, that they had Anton Dolin doing a cabaret which had lasted some time, and that I had taken Joan Gammell home, hence my lateness. She answered, 'She's a nice girl and I'm not surprised you picked her to take home. I've never heard of Anton Dolin, whatever he may be, but I am surprised you got home so early. In my day a ball never finished until five in the morning, then we had beer and bones and were taken home by our chaperones, if they could find us. The fun about chaperones was giving them the slip. I'm sure you and Joan chaperoned each other well!' A wonderful person, my grandmother, always supporting the fight for the liberation of women!

In 1933, on one of my occasional trips to London when a medical student, I was asked by a mutual friend to go to a party with him at Leigh Holman's house in Little Stanhope Street, off the Shepherd's Market area. Leigh Holman was a barrister who had not long been married to a beautiful girl, twelve years younger than him and six months younger than me. She had been born Vivian Hartley at Darjeeling, in India, where her father was in the Indian Cavalry, being stationed among other places at Ootacamund, S. India. Vivian Holman was later to become famous as Vivien Leigh (the spelling of her christian name was changed for 'show' purposes). Vivian had just had baby Suzanne, who was about three months old the first time I met her. The Holmans' house was no distance from University Motors, where I always parked my car when in London. This was the first of several visits I paid to the house in Little Stanhope Street, between 1933 and 1939. Vivian was always charming to me in her enchanting way. Having once met one never forgot her, and she also remembered people of whom she was fond, among whom I flatter myself I was one. She had a great sense of humour and was very considerate to others and, in 1933, much in love with her husband. In London the Holmans were on many visiting lists, including that of the 'Royal' Bairds of Buckingham Palace Mews, so one met them outside their own Shepherd's Market House, Vivian was an aspiring actress, and it was sad to see her life with Leigh Holman slip away because he had to do his law work in his chambers at the Temple and she was gradually becoming better known professionally. This denied Leigh the evenings which he should have been spending with her and their daughter, Suzanne. But she developed first an admiration for Laurence Olivier's acting prowess, and then a passionate love for him which was reciprocated. This made her feel very guilty about her dwindling relationship with Leigh and Suzanne (she was never a maternal type), and about Jill Esmond and Tarquin, Olivier's wife and son. I did not see the Holmans together after 1939 but I met Vivian again in later years.

Final Years at the University
The third, fourth and fifth years of my medical schooling at Aberdeen University were happy and busy ones. The university was fortunate in having chosen Professor Laybourne Stanley Patrick Davidson (Stanley) as Regius Professor of Medicine in 1930. He replaced Professor Sir Ashley Macintosh, a local consultant who had been appointed to the chair many years previously and was not up to date with developments in the medical profession. On the other hand Stanley had shown himself to be an excellent research worker in the Department of Bacteriology at Edinburgh University between 1923 and 1929 when he obtained his MD, his thesis being on the subject of 'Immunisation and antibody reactions: a series of experimental studies'.

When appointed to the Regius Professor of Medicine in Aberdeen at the age of thirty-six in 1930, he was the new type of young and dynamic professor with a research background who expected to develop his department into a teaching school based on, and carrying out, research into the clinical aspects of medicine. An excellent account of Stanley Davidson's life and work has been given by Dr R. Passmore in the *Year Book of the Royal Society of Edinburgh*, 1983. Professor Davidson was president of the Royal College of Physicians of Edinburgh and was Queen's Physician in Scotland. He was knighted in 1955.

My intake of medical students (1930-1935), and Aberdeen University, were fortunate also in having Professor James Learmonth as Regius Professor of Surgery. He, like Stanley Davidson, was a young man when he was appointed to the chair in 1932. He was a Glasgow student who had carried out post-graduate research work on blood groups and on the autonomic nervous system. He specialised in neuro-surgery and was appointed to the staff of the Mayo Clinic in the United States whence he was appointed to Aberdeen University. In 1938 he succeeded Professor Sir David Wilkie as Professor of Surgery at Edinburgh University and took Sandy Slessor, my classmate in Aberdeen, with him as assistant in his new department. With the assistance of Sandy Slessor, Professor Learmonth operated on King George VI in Buckingham Palace in 1949, a lumbar sympathectomy for poor circulation in the lower limbs. The King knighted Professor Learmonth in his (the monarch's) bathroom (Rose 1985), Sandy getting an MVC.

In the mid-1930s about thirty medicaments were essential for the treatment of specific diseases or paleation of symptoms. Among these were insulin and other hormones, quinine and preparations of digitalis, opium and its derivatives, and acetyl salicylic acid (aspirin). Many others were used but were mostly of minor importance or psychological in action, e.g. pink cough medicine or 'tonics'. Hence Professor James Campbell, of the chair of Materia Medica, did not have a very important role to play in our medical education; he taught us how to write prescriptions in Latin and how to use the British Pharmacopoeia. Recent days have seen the development of innumerable medicaments which have specific actions either upon bacterial or viral infections, upon abnormal or cancerous cells or in physiological secretions such as the inhibition of hydrochloric acid secretion in the stomach, thus helping in the treatment of peptic ulceration.

Professor Campbell's best lecture was on the use of alcohol, in which he stressed its depressant effect when drunk in solitude, telling the story of his own experience of shutting himself in his room with a bottle of whisky, drinking it all in two hours and only feeling miserably ill as a result. He made the most of what I considered a boring subject. He was interested in the good name of the medical profession, becoming eventually chairman of the General Medical Council.

The chair of obstetrics and gynaecology was, unfortunately for my year, held by one of the old type of local consultants with a large private practice, who gave his course of lectures and taught at the bedside of his wards. Professor McKerron was a graduate of Aberdeen and had not travelled far or worked much outside 'Aberdeen and twelve miles around', the expression used by Aberdonians themselves to indicate with some pride the parochial nature and self-sufficiency of the town. The 'Howd', as was the inevitable nickname of the Professor of Obstetrics, derived from the expression 'Howdie-wife', or midwife, in the local vernacular, was not a good teacher but he was clinically a shrewd and competent practitioner. He did not try to develop a department of obstetrics, with an adequate staff and research facilities. This was left to his successor, Professor Dougald Baird, a Glasgow graduate and a most dynamic man who put his department well and truly in the limelight of British medicine. With his staff, notably Angus Thomson and a number of social service workers, he investigated the family backgrounds and states of nutrition of the child-bearing population of the city of Aberdeen and many more than twelve miles around. Unfortunately he was not appointed to the university when I was a student, although, through Dougald Baird's co-operation with Stanley Davidson when I was a post-graduate assistant in the Department of Medicine, I had the opportunity to observe his work and the development of his department in the years 1937-39.

Professor Shennan of the Chair of Pathology had been a student of my grandfather, around the turn of the century. We learnt the techniques for carrying out post-mortems and the relationship between the cause of death, almost always well known to the clinician in charge of the case, and the pathological findings. We also spent hours peering down microscopes and learning the cytological appearance of diseased tissues.

Bacteriology was more interesting to me than pathology. Professor Cruikshank was one of the old brigade, but had done a considerable amount of work on the nature of the immunity derived by children, including his own, to tuberculosis. He showed that the acquisition of immunity to the disease depended to a great extent upon the general state of health and nutrition of children, and that this was dependent largely upon environmental sanitation and the parents' knowledge of how best to feed their children. He had also experimented with the production of immunity to TB and inoculation with BCG (Bacillus Calmette-Guerin).

Our teaching in paediatrics was somewhat meagre, being conducted by the consultant paediatrician at the Hospital for Sick Children and in the out-patient department of the Royal Infirmary by the consultant physicians and others, e.g. assistants in the Department of Midwifery.

We had a good course of systematic lectures in orthopaedic surgery delivered by the senior consultant in the subject at the Royal Infirmary, Mr Alex Mitchell. Much practical experience was always available in the out-patient and casualty departments. Orthopaedics is a subject in which great advances have been made in recent years. The development of physiotherapy, with special departments for its practice at most major hospitals, is of the utmost importance in the treatment not only of disabilities due to injuries and arthritic conditions but also to such illnesses as multiple sclerosis, Parkinson's disease and to the after-effects on the neuro-muscular systems of cerebral haemorrhage and embolism. Our orthopaedic training certainly lacked the emphasis which should be given to the practice of physiotherapy.

We were taught how to give simple anaesthetics by the senior anaesthetist, Dr Rose McKenzie, and by Dr Thomas McDonald. This teaching covered the use of chloroform or other gas administered by a mask over the patient's face (the rag and bottle method) and 'gas an oxygen' (nitrous oxide and oxygen) through a Boyle's machine. Most of our practical experience and responsibility in anaesthetics came when we were housemen in the Royal Infirmary, doing casualty or night emergency work.

Forensic medicine was a minor subject as taught to us by Dr Robert Richards, a general practitioner by trade, the police surgeon for the city of Aberdeen and a poor lecturer. This subject is now such a complicated one that it should be dealt with as a full-time post-graduate speciality, and Dr Richards probably taught us all we needed to know on the assumption that most of us were to become general practitioners.

The study of the patient at the bedside was now the most important part of our activities. *Clinical Methods*, first published in 1897, was by far the most important of the volumes I now had to master. 'Case taking' as described in the latest edition by Hutchison and Hunter forms the basis of reaching the diagnosis of what is wrong with the patient, from malingering at the one end to advanced disease at the other. It requires the use of all one's special senses; speech, to interrogate the patient; hearing, to listen to the patient's answers and to interpret correctly the sounds heard through a stethoscope; sight, to assess the patient's general appearance and to see any lesions or abnormalities on the surface of the body or in the retina and optic disc at the back of the eye using an ophthalmoscope or of the eardrum using an auriscope; touch, to determine any abnormality in the size or position of those organs of the body which are capable of being palpated, to ascertain the location and nature of abnormal tumours; to feel the nature of the pulse produced by the heart's beat, or the feel of broken bones rubbing together their fractured surfaces; and smell, to determine the cleanliness of the individual under examination, or any unusual aroma on the breath such as acetone or alcohol. Having followed the outline of interrogation and examination described in *Clinical Methods*, including the analysis of urine and blood which can be easily carried out in the 'side room' of a hospital ward or in the general practitioner's surgery, a very good chance of having reached a definite diagnosis should exist thus leading to the possibility of giving the patient or his relatives or friends a 'prognosis' or forecast of the course of the disease, if indeed such illness exists, and leading to the nature of any treatment required. In the absence of a firm diagnosis it may be necessary to send samples of body fluids to the clinical biochemical department; to the X-ray (different parts of the body) to find out the exact positions of fractured bones, or by administering radio-opaque substances to visualise the nature and extent of gastro-intestinal or intra-cranial abnormalities or lesions in other parts of the body. However, if the case-taking and clinical examination has been as thorough as it should have been, the need for such ancillary biochemical and radiological tests should be kept to a minimum. The excessive use of biochemical laboratories for such tests was often interpreted by the biochemist as a sign of incompetence on the part of the clinician and his housemen, and in some teaching hospitals led to running battles between the two sides.

Since the Second World War the pharmaceutical companies have started to produce drugs, antibiotics, hormones and other therapeutic preparations at an astounding rate. The British National Formulary has to be published very frequently to keep practitioners informed of the nature of these drugs and preparations, many of which can be dangerous and react with other therapeutic substances to produce undesirable interactions. In my days as a houseman or assistant in university medical departments the electron microscope had not been devised; Watson and Crick did not develop the concept of the double helix and deoxyribose nucleic acid (RNA) until 1952, hence the studies of cytology, genetics and genetic engineering and of the nature of the immune system were unknown to us. In fact all these developments have taken place following the establishment of the National Health Service in 1948 by Aneurin Bevan. The present day general practitioner has to learn and practise much more than he had to do in my day of active practice — in fact I believe that he is under much more medico-legal strain than was his predecessor working under the National Health Insurance Act of 1913. He does not, in my opinion, have enough time to spend on each patient in the way expected and outlined in *Clinical Methods*. The gathering of a superficial medical history and of clinical manifestations, plus some biochemical and radiological data, putting them together in a computer-like manner and hoping that a satisfactory diagnosis and outline of treatment will emerge should be shunned in view of its likely inaccuracy. But the poor practitioner has so many patients to see nowadays, not all of them really ill and many wasting his time, that he or she has little alternative.

Having said my say on such matters I find it a relief to be able to report that I was taught in the wards by the methods advocated by *Clinical Methods*; was not worried by a superfluity of new medicines with specific and maybe dangerous actions and side-effects, and that at the end of the summer term in 1935 I qualified MB, ChB (Aberdeen) with much less detailed knowledge than would be required of me in the 1980s. That year I was very glad to win the Anderson Gold Medal for Clinical Medicine, after a searching examination at the bedsides of many patients by the professor and all the senior medical consultants. I had decided that my future was to be a physician rather than a surgeon, and to have as little as possible to do with obstetrics and gynaecology.

CHAPTER 3

Practising as a Doctor

House Physician
During the clinical years 1933 to 1935 every member of my class was no doubt working out in his or her mind what to do on qualification. For some the decision would be relatively easy if they aspired to follow their fathers as general practitioners, others wanted to become consultants in one or other of the branches of the profession. Our professors and the teaching consultants with wards at the Aberdeen Royal Infirmary, Woolmanhill, had also been studying the competence and backgrounds of us, the students. Both Professor Stanley Davidson and Professor James Learmonth had asked me to be their house-physician and house-surgeon respectively. They had both, also, asked A. J. Slessor (Sandy) the same thing. So it was left to Sandy and me to decide which of us started with which professor first, i.e. at the beginning of July 1935, each appointment to be for six months. As I hoped to become a physician and Sandy to be a surgeon, I started with Professor Davidson and he with Professor Learmonth. In those days our families had to pay our tuition and examination fees. For the privilege of living and working in the Residency of ARI at Woolmanhill we were paid at the rate of fifty pounds (£50) per annum. This was a fact which influenced the ability of some students to take a 'house' job following qualification as they wanted to earn more as soon as possible. At this time (1935) to be a houseman in the Royal Infirmary, Edinburgh, a charge of £50 per annum was made for the privilege. On the clinical medicine side Professor Davidson's assistants in the Department of Medicine were John MacMichael, Harold Fullerton and Ian Hill. About fourteen of us housemen and more senior post-graduates lived in the Residency. The faithful Peggy, the Residency maid, saw to it that we were woken in the mornings, made our beds and

PRACTISING AS A DOCTOR

generally kept us up to scratch. Without her we would often have been late for our various ward rounds, clinics, and so on.

The life of a house-physician or house-surgeon was a very busy one, the hours long, often twenty-four hours a day, especially on the surgical side because acute surgical emergencies admitted at night are more frequent than acute medical cases. The major part of one's time was spent in the wards of the professor or consultant to whom one was appointed.

One medical and one surgical ward was on call every day, i.e. one day out of three each houseman was on call for twenty-four hours. The houseman on duty, be he on the medical or surgical side, was primarily responsible for the casualty department. He had to make the decision whether he could cope with a patient himself or should admit the case to the appropriate receiving ward. We used to calculate that our work covered about one hundred and ten hours per seven-day week. However, as the work was fascinating to me and gave me a great deal of happiness, I and most of my colleagues in the Residency never thought of complaining. We were all learning our trade and fifty years ago the opportunity to do so was considered to be a happy affair. At the risk of appearing an old-fashioned 'square', or whatever the expression may be, I cannot understand the reasons for complaint about their working hours so often expressed by present-day housemen, as frequently reported in the press. They work no longer hours than we did, want to work many fewer hours, and are paid a salary at least in four figures sterling per annum. Perhaps they are basically idler than we were and do not believe, as we did with Jerome K. Jerome, that 'it is impossible to enjoy idling thoroughly unless one has plenty of work to do'.

Our time for 'idling' while living in the ARI Residency amounted to about two evenings per seven-day week. We were not allowed to bring any of the opposite sex, including nurses, into the building and, as I remember, few of us at that particular time of our lives had any time for girlfriends.

One evening three of us had been to Harry Gordon's music hall show and had heard an electrified guitar being played by one of the male artistes. About 3 a.m. the next morning I was awakened by the casualty officer on duty saying he had admitted an 'acute abdomen' to my ward, i.e. Prof. Learmonth's ward. The patient was the guitar player, who undoubtedly had an acute abdominal condition which I could not diagnose. So I called Gordon Bruce, the senior surgeon on the professor's team, who reluctantly came to the hospital. He also could not decide what was the cause of the trouble but it was obvious that we had to find out by opening the abdomen. The man was suffering from acute pancreatitis, a condition often found among heavy drinkers. There being nothing positive to do in such a case Mr Bruce inserted a large drain to the pancreatic area and closed the wound, asking me to keep an eye on the patient when he came round from the anaesthetic. I returned to bed again about 5 a.m. I was awakened by the staff nurse on duty who I could see was very worried, as she had every reason to be. I found the guitarist, with his wound split open and considerable amounts of small intestine hanging out, chasing a junior nurse round the ward. With the help of the night porter and nursing staff I anaesthetised him on his bed, using ether, returned his intestines to their rightful place, sewed him up with the drain still *in situ* and kept him under heavy sedation with omnopon/scopolamine for the next twelve hours. He then started having *delirium tremens,* which lasted some days, but was controlled by chloral hydrate and potassium bromide. The delirium stopped, his wound healed and the pancreatitis subsided. He walked out of the ward after three weeks, as if he had never been ill but he was an extremely lucky man and I often wondered how long he went on playing his guitar.

It is important to emphasise the amount we learnt about our job and proper attitude to patients from the ward sisters and their senior nurses. In ward five, Professor Davidson's ward, Sister Clark was outstanding. She taught me more about the practical aspects of dealing with bedridden patients than did the teaching staff. Sister Clark knew much more about the diagnosis and treatment of patients than I did, but had to pretend that I was her superior in this sphere. From time to time she would tactfully admit to me that she did not know if the professor really knew what he was about, and then give me her own views, derived from many years of nursing experience, which included playing off the immature views of the house-physician against those of the resident, assistant consultant and professor, all of which might vary in a different case. I remember the occasion when neither the professor, the assistant consultant, Dr John MacMichael, the registrar or myself could reach a diagnosis in the case of a woman aged about forty years, who had been admitted at the request of her general practitioner and had been in the ward for nearly a week. She was quite deeply jaundiced but she only complained of weakness, no abdominal pain. Clinical examination was negative, liver not enlarged, radiologically she did not appear to have gallstones, and such liver function tests as were then available to use were equivocal. At the morning ward round, Professor Davidson wracked his and our brains as to the causation of her jaundice. At last he turned to Sister Clark and said, 'Sister, what do we do?' She replied, 'Get Professor McKerron to see her.' As this was the 'Howd' why should he be asked to see her? However, he kindly came over from his own ward, stood at the end of the bed and listened to the case history. He asked if she was pregnant and I had to admit I did not know. Nor did the Professor or John MacMichael, but Sister said she was between two and three months pregnant, and in the past had had four children. The 'Howd' looked at the women again for a moment and took Stanley into the side room where he said, 'She has acute yellow atrophy of her liver and will be dead within three weeks.' She had, and she was! A good example of failure to obtain all the facts about a case at the case-taking stage! We never found out what was the cause of this case of acute massive necrosis of the liver.

While I was house physician to Stanley Davidson, he and Harold Fullerton were working on the causation of the anaemia which was particularly prevalent at the time in Aberdeen among young women and mothers of several children, probably due to the economic depression of the early 1930s. They published a number of papers on the subject, showing it to be of nutritional origin due to dietary iron deficiency, which was easily treated by the administration of dried ferrous sulphate 200 mg three times a day, after food to avoid gastric irritation, continued until the woman's dietary stores of iron were replenished and coupled with nutritional education.

On several occasions while I was Stanley's house-physician, patients were admitted with a febrile disease coupled with signs of jaundice and haemorrhage into mucous membrane and the subcutaneous tissues. John MacMichael and Ian Hill were set to work on this unusual syndrome and it was eventually diagnosed as Weil's disease, caused by infection from a spirochaete, *Leptospira icterohaemorrhagiae*. The patients were all fish workers at the Aberdeen harbour, and the source of the infection was traced to rats in the fishmarket which carried the germ. Once this phase of the research had been complete by the Department of Medicine at the university, the prevention became the responsibility of the public health department of the city.

Everyone in the active department of medicine which Stanley had developed since his advent in Aberdeen was doing research work and he soon began to direct my attention, although I was only a house-physician learning to practise my profession, towards a line of research in which he was becoming interested. He had the capacity to be able to identify areas of illness about which he felt more knowledge should be gained in order to help the profession to give better service to patients. The area where he felt I could start to do some work and thinking of my own was that of peptic ulceration of the stomach and duodenum.

A very large number of cases of gastric and duodenal ulcers was being admitted to his wards, both on the male and female side. They tended to be long-term patients who occupied beds for a number of weeks or months and this had an adverse effect on the numbers on the waiting list for admission to hospital. Such ulcer patients were often admitted as medical emergencies due to acute blood loss either vomited up or passed by the bowel. Stanley had already started to use a method for treating bleeding ulcers developed in Denmark by a friend of his, Meulengracht, which consisted of giving a diet including finely minced beef, chicken, tripe or other sources of animal protein, the object being to reduce the amount of acidity in the stomach. and duodenum and thus allow not only the healing of the ulcer but also to provide a start to the process of treating the anaemia suffered by the patients, which was of greater or lesser amount due to the amount of blood loss. Most of these acute cases required blood transfusion in the first place and it was the houseman's job to find a suitable blood donor from among the patient's relatives or friends and cross-match the available blood with that of the patient. In those days a blood transfusion service and blood banks did not exist. Before the introduction of the Meulengracht diet, the conservative treatment of peptic ulcer was to give a milk-based diet after the pattern developed by Hurst in the United Kingdom or Sippey in the United States.

Small doses of a mild sedation such as phenobarbitone were also given to allay the tension often suffered by peptic ulcer patients. Not all such cases were admitted as emergencies, in fact most of them came from the waiting list on which they had been placed by the general practitioners because of the intractable dyspepsia from which they suffered.

Stanley asked me to pay particular attention to the case histories of all patients admitted to the ward with symptoms or signs of gastric or duodenal ulcer with particular reference to their family and employment backgrounds, and to make certain of the diagnosis, together with the site of the ulcer in the stomach or duodenum with the aid of radiologists, whom he asked to help me. He also gave me the responsibility of calling in surgeons when necessary to consider the need for operation to stop massive haemorrhages or to perform some of the definitive operations than carried out with the object of reducing gastric acidity the commonest at that time being gastro-enterostomy or partial gastrectomy. In respect of surgical co-operation I relied largely on Sandy Slessor, house-surgeon to Professor Learmonth, for making arrangements which would fit in well with the surgical programme. Learmonth and his senior registrar, Norman Logie, were both interested in gastric surgery and co-operated readily. It then became my responsibility to follow up the cases treated surgically and compare the results with those of our own cases treated purely medically. In addition to interrogation of the patients and their radiological examination I carried out fractional test meals on all cases diagnosed as suffering from gastric and duodenal ulcers. After a few weeks this approach to the nature and causation of peptic ulcers began to yield some results in the way of sex incidence, ratio of gastric to duodenal ulcers, various connections between occupation, diets consumed and stresses and strains of life upon the ratio between the two types of ulcer after cancer of the stomach had been excluded, and the response to treatment in terms of gastric acidity determined by fractional test meals conducted from the fasting state. Research into these factors was continued by me until the outbreak of war and the final conclusions will be reported later in this book.

But acute haemorrhages from gastric and duodenal ulcers were not the only sorts of emergencies we had in medical wards. Comas caused by diabetes, due either to abnormally high or low blood sugar levels, were frequent. Hyperpyrexia due to such diseases as meningitis, typhoid fever or malaria were not uncommon and had to be diagnosed before they were or were not sent to the hospital for infectious diseases. Acute lobar pneumonia also presented itself in emergency form, and after correct diagnosis became the responsibility of the patient's stamina and the competence of the nursing staff if they were to survive prior to the availability of antibiotics.

Two cases of lobar pneumonia gave Sister Clark the opportunity to teach me a lesson I have never forgotten. The patients were recruits about twenty years old, from the Gordon Highlanders' barracks in Aberdeen, and had been screened off from the rest of the ward together. They were not allowed any visitors because they were very seriously ill. Two days after their admission I noticed talk coming from behind the screens and found two clergymen, one a Presbyterian minister and the other a Roman Catholic priest. As the patients were so ill and not allowed visitors, I asked the clergymen to retire, which they did reluctantly, as I found later to complain to Sister. Within half an hour she had explained to me that, if a patient had a religious faith of any sort, not confined only to Christendom, he or she should never be denied the presence of their priest of whatever denomination, particularly if they were extremely ill or dying.

Another emergency was admitted one day, a potential male suicide who had swallowed about a pint of neat carbolic acid previously, two hours. Although I knew carbolic acid to be corrosive, the short length of time since its ingestion and the presence of an active gag reflex encouraged me to pass a stomach tube and wash out his stomach with saline. He made a good recovery but was a very ungrateful patient.

House Surgeon

At the end of December 1935 Sandy Slessor and I changed over our appointments and I became house surgeon to Professor James Learmonth. He had on his firm on ward one Mr Gordon Bruce (mentioned above) as consultant and Mr Norman Logie as assistant surgeon and registrar. The professor's main interest was neuro-surgery, particularly that of the autonomic nervous system. He was also a competent general surgeon, particularly in the field of gastro-enterology. Gordon Bruce specialised in surgery of the thyroid gland but was also a good general surgeon. Norman Logie was a first-class general surgeon in the making.

By 1936 our knowledge of the anatomy and physiology of the central and autonomic nervous systems was sufficiently good to enable lesions such as cerebral tumours or malfunctions such as spasm of peripheral arteries leading to intermittent clandication (pain in the extremities due to constricted blood vessel) to be diagnosed quite accurately provided the clinical methods described by Hutchison and Hunter were followed and accurately interpreted. The house surgeon had the privilege of taking the case history and making the first clinical examination and, in writing up the notes for the chief, he had to make a first attempt at reaching a conclusion, suggest any additional procedures which might be necessary such as lumbar puncture to ascertain the pressure, appearance and biochemical composition of the fluid within the membrane surrounding the spinal core, and brain, or in the introduction of air into the cavities within the brain to enable X-ray pictures to show up any abnormalities. Such case-taking and clinical work fascinated me and frequently the professor agreed with my tentative diagnosis. While we could be accurate in locating a lesion it was more difficult in some cases to be sure of its nature. For instance on one occasion the diagnosis of a space-occupying tumour at the base of the brain between the cerebellum and brain stem was made. The patient was a boy aged about five years. We had a suspicion from the case history which indicated that the growth was increasing in size rather fast, and from the age of the patient, that the tumour might be malignant (cancerous). As radiation therapy was not yet sufficiently developed and would be dangerous to the vital areas around the location of the lesion, the only solution was to operate, hoping it would be non-cancerous. When the bone-flat at the posterior of the skull had been turned down and the coverings of the brain retracted, the tumour was exactly where we expected it to be but it was unfortunately malignant. Nothing remained to be done but to close up the cerebral membrane, bony skull and scalp. The patient lived for a few months before his inevitable death. The use of expensive modern equipment such as scanners would not have located the sight of the lesion any more accurately than we could do at that time by careful and accurate clinical examination.

For a period of three weeks a number of Professor Learmonth's patients suffered from infections of the skin at the site of abdominal scars. Fortunately this infection never affected our scalp incisions, possibly because the scalp has such an abundant blood supply and normally heals well and quickly. In view of the abdominal skin infection, Professor Cruikshank's staff from the Bacteriology Department was called in to check our autoclaves, the theatre air and ventilation systems. Nothing in the way of pathogenic bacteria was found to match the Staphylococcus cultured from the wounds. So the theatre sister and her staff were swabbed — still nothing! Then I swabbed the professor's throat and he swabbed mine and there they were in my tonsils! The next morning my tonsils and adenoids had been dissected out by Jack Otty, the senior ear, nose and throat surgeon in Kepplestone Nursing Home and I was back working in the theatre in four days, my throat sore but not as sore as my windpipe which the anaesthetist had damaged with his endotracheal tube. But we did not have any more infected abdominal wounds!

Little by little I developed some surgical technique and confidence, through experience gained mainly from general abdominal surgery and more specialised neuro-surgery and operations on the thyroid gland. This learning process continued until July 1936, when Professor Learmonth was asked by Mr A. R. D. Pattison, the neuro-surgeon in the Newcastle-upon-Tyne and Durham areas, if he could suggest a locum for his neuro-surgical registrar, Clerk-Maxwell by name and a grandson of the physicist, who had to take some months' holiday for family reasons. Professor Learmonth recommended me for the job and I went to Newcastle early in August 1936, after taking three weeks' leave following a hectic year in Aberdeen Royal Infirmary.

Neuro-Surgical Registrar, General Hospital, Newcastle

I found Mr Pattison (Patt) a delightful man with whom to work. He was a very competent neuro-surgeon but preferred the central nervous system as his major field of activity, tending to leave work on the involuntary system (nervous) to the neurologists and cardio-vascular experts. His wards and out-patients department, for which I was responsible, were in the General Hospital, Wingrove Road, Newcastle. This rather elderly building, known as 'The Wingrove', housed three very different specialised units, neuro-surgery, plastic surgery and thoracic surgery. The plastic surgeon was Mr William Wardle and the thoracic surgeon, an ex-pupil and house surgeon to the famous Grey Turner, was Mr George Mason, who had an Edinburgh graduate, Andrew Logan, as his registrar at that time. On my arrival I was surprised to find that Mr Wardle's firm did not have a registrar and that it was my privilege, pleasure and duty to fill that appointment, as well as the primary one of neuro-surgery. I soon found that this was a valuable adjunct to my main job, as Bill Wardle, after Sir Harold Gilles, was one of the best plastic surgeons in the country at that time. He had also done some original surgical trials on young children suffering from cleft palates. This was surgery at its most delicate, requiring patience and perseverance with very fine cat-gut sutures, using tiny semi-circular needles and fine forceps to perform. Bill Wardle placed the greatest part of the success of these pharyngoplatics with the elocutionist who followed up all his patients. She was a wonderfully patient person, carrying out what she called palato-pharyngeal physiotherapy! This work was all carried out in the Babies Hospital in Newcastle, then under the direction of the very well-known paediatrician, Dr J. C. Spence.

Patt and I, and his trusty theatre staff, 'cracked many a skull' together and visited Sunderland General Hospital to operate there about once a month. For the first several weeks of my stay in Newcastle I found it impossible to take a case history without a nurse to act as interpreter. The 'Geordie' language is more incomprehensible to the 'foreigner', but pleasanter to listen to than the Gorbals Glaswegian noise. After a while I began to realise that 'hinney' means 'my dear' and not 'get the hell out of here', when shouted at me in a loud voice, in response to the suggestion 'what are you complaining about?' I became very attached to Newcastle and the Geordies.

George Mason and Andrew Logan became firm friends of mine. The Masons lived in the Jesmond area, and in their house I met on a personal, rather than a hospital basis, many colleagues including Joan Miller, the young lady anaesthetist who did the difficult anaesthetic work for Bill Wardle's babies. She was a good physician as well as a good anaesthetist, and gave me some comfort helping me with a patient from whom I was unsuccessfully trying to remove his prostate gland, when she said, 'Bad luck, it is malignant. The last time I saw this happen was two weeks ago when I was giving up a "dope" for Mr ——. He left his patient with a surgical suprapubic cystostomy.' Mr —— was one of the Wingrove's senior surgical consultants, so I left my patient with a suprapubic cystostomy also.

Voyage as a Ship's Surgeon: December 1936 to May 1937

While I was working in Newcastle it had been agreed by Professor Davidson and me that I would return to Aberdeen to take up a post of assistant in the Department of Medicine. He considered that I should first take a voyage as a ship's surgeon to the Far East. Such a voyage would give me a good rest from the exacting work I had been doing in Aberdeen and Newcastle since the middle of 1935. Stanley was also very keen that I should visit any hospitals in the ports we would visit and there try to ascertain the prevalence of peptic ulcer among the in-patients, as we had started to do in Aberdeen when I was his house physician. What he wanted to know was the ethnic origins, age and sex incidence, ratio of gastric to duodenal ulcers and the occupations of the patients. I kept a very detailed diary of the voyage and a separate set of records of the data on peptic ulceration.

I joined the ship in Hamburg and we sailed for the Far East from Rotterdam on 24 December 1936. I was to be surgeon on the S.S. *Teucer* of Alfred Holt's Blue Funnel Line. We anchored off Port Said on 5 January 1937 and I had a talk with the port medical officer, who had qualified at London University (Guy's Hospital) about peptic ulcers in Egyptians and Arabs, a subject which did not interest him. There was not enough time to go to Cairo on my search for ulcer data. We sailed from Port Said on 6 January and our next stop was at Port Sudan early on 9 January — a very hot spot without a hospital, only government buildings and the Red Sea Hotel. Our next port of call was Penang, in the Federated Malay States. I saw the tip of Adam's Peak, Ceylon, on 20 January. We anchored in the roads off Georgetown, Penang, on 25 January 1937.

In Penang I visited the hospital and got some information on peptic ulceration. It was a fine building with three blocks, five hundred beds in all, first, second and third class according to fees paid. The first class wing (fifty beds) was mostly single rooms mainly occupied by Europeans and wealthy Malays and

Chinese; the second class (five or ten beds to a small ward) was also for private patients of more limited means; and the third class (300 beds in open male and female wards) was for non-fee-paying patients. The theatres and X-ray plant was very modern. The hospital grounds were spacious and surrounded by a race track, golf course, and polo field. The hospital was run by four doctors of the Colonial Medical Service, routine but infrequent visits being paid by consultants from Kuala Lumpur, Ipoh or Singapore.

I found that the Alfred Holt Blue Funnel M.V. *Sarpedon* was also in port. I went to the Runnymede Hotel for tea and the Eastern and Oriental Hotel for drinks later. The whole island seemed to be overrun with the *Sarpendon*'s two hundred passengers. I also visited the 'Snake Temple' where I was told unofficially that the green pitt vipers had had their poison fangs removed. We sailed at 7.30 p.m. in the middle of my first tropical thunderstorm.

On 26 January we dropped anchor at Port Swettenham on the Klang River at 1.30 p.m. As we were due to sail at 7 p.m. I had no time to visit the hospital in Kuala Lumpur, thirty miles inland. Early on the morning of 27 January we passed Raffles Island and anchored in the Singapore Roads. I went ashore at Hilton Pier, getting soaked in the process due to rough water and a heavy shower, so went to John Little's to get another white suit. I went to Raffles Hotel for lunch and then to the hospital, which is arranged on the same lines as the one in Penang. The staff were not inclined to show me round and let me look at their records in the afternoon (siesta time) and I made a date to visit them in the morning on our return voyage. We left Singapore for Hong Kong on 28 January. We had taken on a number of deck passengers for Hong Kong and Shanghai, one of whom I found to be suffering from the wet form of beri-beri and admitted him to the sick bay. As my dispensary did not contain any vitamin preparations I gave him plenty of yeast, fruit (papaya) and green vegetables and tincture of digitalis which he took under protest. We anchored in Kowloon bay and discharged some dangerous cargo (methydol) into lighters and then went alongside Holt's Wharf on the Kowloon side, and were tied up by 7.45 p.m. on 2 February 1937. I spent most of the next day examining new firemen who had signed on and saying goodbye to my own boy, Ho Ling, who had looked after my cabin, clothes and the dispensary room from Hamburg to Hong Kong.

On the evening of 3 February I went over to Victoria Island by sampan and met Maidie Gordon, who had been Maidie Gairdner from Skelmorlie, and her husband, Vyner Gordon, who was the senior engineer in charge of the Peak Railway, which is a rack railway running from downtown Hong Kong to the col between Victoria Peak and Mount Cameron. On 4 February I visited the teaching hospital of the University of Hong Kong, on the west side of the peak, run by the Colonial Medical Service. The professor of medicine was on leave but I got a considerable amount of data about peptic ulceration. On 5 February we were off again for Shanghai. My beri-beri case seemed to be holding his own.

On 6 February we were in the Formosa Straits surrounded by Chinese fishing vessels. The weather was becoming cold (55° F). My new 'batman' was called Ng Pak, not easy to pronounce. The beri-beri case died the night before and we had to go into quarantine at Holt's Wharf in Shanghai, downstream from the famous Bund in the International Settlement area of the city. The quarantine officer came on board promptly and cleared the ship so we got the 'yellow jack' down and on with the working of cargo.

We had three days in Shanghai and I had a good opportunity to obtain the information I wanted from the hospital which looks after the expatriates in the International Settlements and also the local Chinese, Korean and other Far Eastern ethnic groups collected in the city. I also met by chance a school friend by the name of Ian Macrae who worked for Butterfield and Swire, the Holt's agents. He took me around the town; the race course and the polo club, Palace and Cathay Hotels, Szechuan Road, Broadway Mansions across the Suchow Creek, and Maxime's nightclub. It was Chinese New Year and all the main streets were beautifully decorated and lit up.

We sailed on 10 February for Darien, where the temperature was $-10°$ C. The hospital at Darien dealt mainly with the staff of the Trans-Siberian railway and the doctors did not seem to know anything about peptic ulcers.

The *Sarpedon* arrived in Darien just as we left. She was filling her cool-chamber (freezer) with a cargo of pheasants! The

Japanese authorities did not allow cameras ashore in the Darien peninsula, which appeared to be heavily fortified.

From Darien we sailed for Kobe in Japan on 15 February. We passed Quelpart Island with its Mount Auckland looking very fine in the Yellow Sea on our port side, round Yaku Shima, one of the southernmost islands of Japan, and along the coast of Kyushu and Shikoku to Kobe at the eastern end of the Inland Sea, reached on 18 February, with the volcanic island of Iwoga-Shima to starboard. It is reputed to be one of the island craters up which suicides climb before throwing themselves in.

In Kobe, on the main island of Honshu, which we reached on 18 February, I ordered a set of coffee cups in fine painted china and some shirts to be collected on our homeward voyage.

The traffic in Kobe was very bad, controlled by policemen with a board across their shoulders; when the board is across the traffic the cars, rickshaws and bicycles are supposed to stop. I took this to mean that pedestrians could then walk across the road but found this was not so and in three minutes I was in the local gaol. On account of all the anti-British feeling in Japan at that time (1937) it took the consul twelve hours to get me out. I celebrated my release, which the chief engineer had helped to organise, by going to a film, unnamed in my diary, but with Joan Bennett and Cary Grant as the main actors, followed by dinner at a restaurant called the Oriental Grill — good oysters, a mixed grill, ice-cream and coffee for three yen. The chief engineer's nickname in these parts is Fuji Yama San, on account of his bald head.

The hospital at Kobe did not have a qualified doctor who spoke enough English to discuss the question of the incidence of peptic ulceration in the population or its hospital prevalence, so I gave up trying on that subject and looked around the hospital. I was not impressed.

I had many Japanese coolies coming to the ship's dispensary with small cuts and bruises, feeling very sorry for themselves. It seems odd that men who are ready to get into a torpedo or commit suicide on small provocation should feel so badly about very minor injuries.

We sailed from Kobe on 22 February and reached Yokohama on the twenty-third. On 24 February a coolie fell from the coaming of No. 9 hatch right down to the orlop deck. He broke his jaw in three places, dislocated his right femur and fractured his left femur. He was unconscious and I managed to get him onto a hatch board as a stretcher, then onto a ship's stretcher and over the side into a lorry which took us to the general hospital. After I put on Japanese slippers I was allowed into the building, which had an antique X-ray set. Nobody spoke any English, but they wanted to keep my stretcher, and I had to get the Butterfield and Swire representative to retrieve it. No question about peptic ulceration there!

At 7.30 a.m. on 28 February we were at Otaru. The doctors and authorities were very strict here, having a full muster of the crew and ship-wide search for opium. The local population are very keen on winter sports and we could see a ski-jump built just behind the town. There was plenty of snow, and I watched some downhill and cross-country races on skis.

From Otaru I badly wanted to get to Sapporo, twelve miles away, where, I had been told in the UK, work was being done in the University Hospital on peptic ulceration. The local police said I could not go outside the port area for security reasons. I climbed a steep conical-shaped hill to a house on the top, the British Consulate. There I found a very elderly Englishman and a Japanese woman, also elderly. When I addressed him he at first replied in Japanese, apologised and then told me in English that I could not go to Sapporo because my passport did not have the correct visa. Yes, the Sapporo University had a good medical school but he was not in touch with the town by telephone. So my best chance to get information on the prevalence of peptic ulceration in Japan was shattered!

Eventually we sailed from Otaru on 4 March 1937 bound for Yokohama via Hakodate again. We were now loading a mixed cargo for UK. The weather in the Tsugaru Strait was extremely bad and the strait very treacherous, but we reached Hakodate without casualties. The 'Old Man' said he had never seen such bad weather hereabouts.

By 8 March we were back in Yokohama and stayed there until 12 March. I visited the main Yokohama hospital where I got a little information about ulcers. It seems that the doctors have difficulty differentiating gastric from duodenal ulcers due to poor clinical case-taking and bad radiography, but they treat cases of haematamesis and melaema by feeding a fishpaste-based diet on the same principle as that used by Meulengracht.

PRACTISING AS A DOCTOR

We reached Nagoya on 13 March. Its only claim to fame is a beautiful view of Fuji Yama. On 24 March we were back in Kobe. The Japanese ship *Heian Maru* was in port being cleaned up to take His Imperial Majesty Prince Chichibu to Canada on his way to the Coronation of King George VI.

On 18 March we met the yellow mud of the Yangtse River fifty miles out at sea. We tied up alongside Holt's Wharf again in the afternoon and I was invited to dine in the Butterfield and Swire mess that evening. Ian Macrae was very excited as his younger brother Duncan was playing in the Calcutta Cup rugby match at Murrayfield next Saturday, his third Scottish cap. We sailed on 20 March for a short stop in Hong Kong, but were fog-bound outside Typhoon Bay until 24 March. I managed to meet the Vyner Gordons for drinks at the Hong Club annex and at the Hong Kong Hotel before dining at the Gloucester Hotel. The mother ship, HMS *Medway*, and her group of submarines, a cruiser and some destroyers were in port, also the Canadian Pacific *Empress of Britain*.

On the way to Singapore I found some of the Chinese firemen's food put out today on a hatch cover — many sorts of filleted fish, shrimps, sea anemones, cabbage, soya bean cake, Chinese turnip, snails and other oddments. The chief cook was making a 'poe' (pie) and offered me a piece with the remark, 'All same plenty good master. Plenty much better when chow more dry — plenty more smell, more taste, more better.' I only managed one mouthful!

On 29 March one of the firemen reported sick with a cough and I thought he had pulmonary tuberculosis. Next morning I took him to the Singapore General Hospital, where my patient was admitted by a pleasant Malay doctor, who handed me on to an English physician. He showed me round the hospital, run on the same lines as the one in Penang. He made the hospital records available to me and gave his own impression that the Straits Chinese suffer from peptic ulcer much more than Malays, and that gastric ulcer is less common than duodenal ulcers in both nationalities. The figures I acquired from the records confirmed his views.

The captain and I went to Raffles for a beer, saw a film called 'The Thin Man' and back to Raffles for dinner. Another evening I went to see the film 'Sunshine Susie' starring Jack Hulbert and dined at Raffles with the doctor from the *Perseus*, another Blue Funnel ship. We went on to the 'New World' dance hall and bar. The girls were beautiful, mostly Chinese/Malay half-castes, but too expensive for both of us as we were broke — one Singapore dollar for four dances!

We arrived at Port Swettenham for twelve hours on 4 April, then on to Penang. Went up Penang Hill to see the sunset and saw a heavy thunderstorm over the mainland beyond Butterworth. The German battleship *Emden* was in the Malacca Straits that day. We sailed for Colombo on 6 April, where we arrived on 11 April at 6 a.m. and sailed again at 7 p..m. for Port Tewfik and the Suez Canal. On 14 April we were in serious trouble due to a fire which started in No. 1 hold, flames erupting round the hatch coamings and out of the ventilators. The fire started in cargo composed of copra, barrels of latex, timber and coconut matting and spread to No. 2 hold. The captain ordered the hold to be filled with steam, which controlled the fire and smoke but some of the latex drums exploded, and the captain had to decide to return to Colombo. When we reached that port it was found necessary to flood the forward holds with sea water, thus settling the ship on the bottom of the harbour and extinguishing the fire. I had been busy treating burns, shock, various minor injuries and inhaled smoke, so it was a pleasant feeling to be inside the harbour about twenty yards from the breakwater. HMS *Norfolk* was also in the harbour.

As I was expected to be back working in the Medicine Department of Aberdeen University by the end of May 1937, Professor Davidson managed to arrange with the Blue Funnel company that I be transferred to the MV *Sarpedon,* now in Colombo. Her MO was not averse to a straight swap, so I took over from him, including the two hundred passengers. I soon found out why Dr Tobin was glad to get away from their numerous complaints, seldom serious. One advantage was that I could make a little money in fees. I removed one acute appendix on the voyage home, in the Indian Ocean, near Aden, with the help of a good theatre staff and 'rag and bone' ether. The *Sarpedon* went straight home with a short sightseeing stop at Aden, Jeddah and Port Tewfik for Cairo. Then back to Liverpool and up to Aberdeen by 24 May 1937.

Medical Research 1937 to 1939
(a) Peptic Ulceration

I was assistant in the Department of Medicine, University of Aberdeen, from June 1937 until the autumn of 1938 when Stanley became Regius Professor of Medicine in the University of Edinburgh. He was kind enough to take me to Edinburgh where I became Carnegie Teaching Fellow in the Department of Medicine at the University of Edinburgh and Clinical Tutor in the Edinburgh Royal Infirmary and remained so until the beginning of the Second World War. During both these appointments my research work was concerned with the causation, prognosis and treatment of peptic ulcer. I also gave lectures to the senior students on these subjects. It required me to carry out ward rounds with third-year students and to introduce them to case-taking at the bedside.

My first research activity was to assemble the data I had collected on the nature of peptic ulceration in the Orient. Then I followed up the condition of 435 patients admitted to two medical wards of the Aberdeen Royal Infirmary between the years 1927 to 1936 inclusive. In all, 387 (89 per cent) of these patients were successfully traced and examined between two and twelve years after their discharge from hospital. The overall objectives were to assess the relative results of medical and surgical treatment of the condition and the frequency of relapse; to compare the distribution of gastric and duodenal ulcers between males and females; to ascertain the hospital prevalence of peptic ulcer within the United Kingdom; and the geographical distribution of gastric and duodenal ulcers in different parts of the world.

The theory that devitalised gastric or duodenal ulcers mucous membrane were prevented from healing and further eroded by the strong hydrochloric acid (HCl) content of the gastric juice had been held since the early days of the twentieth century. Sir Arthur Hurst in England and Dr B. W. Sippy in the United States claimed that complete neutralisation of all the secreted HCl by the stomach during waking hours was achieved when patients were put on a strict dietary regime of hourly feeds of milk with intermediate doses of alkalis, atropine and olive oil. Professor Davidson was doubtful about these claims and suggested that I develop a method of checking them.

Thus in the months from June 1937 to May 1938 I was engaged in trying to determine the family background, age, sex and geographical distribution of gastric and duodenal ulcers in Britain and other parts of the world and in assessing the ability to control gastric acidity in cases of peptic ulcer by means of different dietary regime. New techniques such as determination of free and total gastric HCl at hourly intervals over twenty-four-hour periods had to be developed. The result of all this research was published in full between 1939 and 1941, the delays in some instances being due to the outbreak of the Second World War. A brief summary of the most important findings is as follows:

1. Published data indicated that the ratio of duodenal to gastric ulcer among patients admitted to hospital or private nursing homes varied from 1 to 1 in London, 2 to 1 in Peking, 3 to 1 in Leeds, 4 to 1 in Paris and 8 to 1 in Glasgow, New York and Boston. In Yokohama the few data for Japanese showed the ratio to be 3 to 1. In Singapore, for Chinese patients the ratio was 3 to 1 but among Malays it was 1 to 1. The sex incidence of peptic ulceration (duodenal plus gastric) was remarkably constant in Caucasian races living in their own countries, being approximately 3.5 males to one female. The same ratio for Japanese was 2 to 1 and for Chinese in Peking 3 to 1. For Federated Malay States (FMS) Chinese the figure was 2 to 1 and for Malaya 1 to 1.

2. Neurologists and neuro-surgeons had noted an association between nervous lesions or psychological stress and duodenal ulcer. A nervous stress factor in the causation of duodenal ulcer would help to explain the differences in the worldwide ratio between gastric ulcers and duodenal ulcers in all geographic areas except London and Leeds, and also, the observed differences in sex ratio. It was well known that the Chinese worked much harder and, through their business acumen, were likely to place themselves under more mental or psychological stress than the Malays. The Chinese, either in the Federated Malay States or Peking, were likely to suffer less stress than the men in big European or United States cities. The consumption of physically rough or highly spiced food could well be a factor likely to damage the gastric mucosa of orientals more than Caucasians and thus reduce the ratio of duodenal to gastric ulcers. With due respect to the ladies in the first three decades of the twentieth century, before the campaign for freedom for women had achieved much success, and before the advent of the female executives, politicians or Prime Ministers, the brunt of the responsibility and stresses and

strains of daily life rested with men. This would explain the predominance of duodenal ulcer in the male sex. Case histories in duodenal ulcer patients indicated an hereditary factor in males more often than in females. I summarised the conclusions of the research as follows (British Medical Journal, 1941, ii, 780):

Two different sets of factors are at work in the causation of peptic ulceration. These can be called 'D' factors, leading to duodenal ulcer, and 'G' factors, resulting in gastric ulcer. The 'D' factors are usually inherited, but may be aggravated or even originated by mental stress and anxiety. They are active most frequently in the third decade of life, and appear to be psychosomatic in character. The 'G' factors, on the other hand, are not inherited, occur throughout life more or less uniformly from the second to the sixth decade, and lead to local trauma of the gastric mucosa. The sum of 'D' and 'G' factors causes peptic ulceration approximately three times as often in males as in females (in Caucasian countries).

The only way the low incidence of cases of duodenal ulcer reported from hospitals in London and Leeds could be explained was that in those cities patients with uncomplicated duodenal ulcer were treated more frequently as out-patients or in their homes by general practitioners than in other cities. This was an unsatisfactory conclusion.

Early in 1938 I joined a small group of gastro-enterologists interested particularly in peptic ulceration. The meetings at the Middlesex Hospital were organised by Dr Harold Rogers of St Bartholomew's Hospital, the object being to learn how best to use the semi-flexible gastroscope which had only recently come into general use. We practised upon ourselves how best to pass the instrument into the stomach so as to get the best direct view of the gastric and pre-pyloric mucous membrane and familiarise ourselves with its appearance in the healthy state. Then we carried out trials by introducing various substances into the stomach through a Ryle's tube which we passed before inserting the gastroscope. Normal foodstuffs could not be used even in purified form as they obstructed our view of the mucosa. However, the effects of clear liquids could be investigated in this manner and we were relieved to find out that neat whisky, brandy or gin did not make the mucous membrane even blush. However, sticky liqueurs such as Cointreau or Grenadine produced a generalised reddening of the stomach lining. We also noticed that the small white particles from an emulsion of insoluble aspirin were surrounded by bright red areas of inflammation, as were particles of mustard, pepper and curry powder. This gave a lead to the type of substance which could start the process of devitalisation of the mucosa which, by the action of the acid and pepsin-containing gastric juice could go on to produce gastric erosions and eventually ulcers of the stomach. It was little wonder that the Chinese and Japanese had a higher ratio of gastric to duodenal ulcers than their European and American counterparts!

It is here that the following important point must be made. Up to now the research which I reported in full in the medical journals was concerned only with data derived from hospitalised patients. Were the conclusions drawn concerning the relative incidence of duodenal to gastric ulcers, or the sex ratios reported, applicable to whole populations? The London figures indicated that conclusions should not be drawn about the overall prevalence of peptic ulcer from the hospital statistics recorded. In the future, particularly when I was working in the Colonial Medical Service in Nigeria, I always tried to determine the prevalence of any disease or abnormal state of nutrition as it occurred in complete populations or in representative samples thereof.

The development of the twenty-four-hour method of determining the free and total HCl in the stomach clearly demonstrated that the Hurst and Sippy diets fell far short of the complete neutralisation of all acid during waking hours claimed for them in cases of uncomplicated peptic ulcer. This we found to be due to the rapidity with which the milk, when given in five or ten ounce amounts hourly or two hourly, together with atrophine and alkalis, was emptied from the stomach. Five ounces of milk given by continuous drip during the day controlled the free gastric acidity but this was followed by a high secretion of free HCl at night. We found that the best means of reducing free HCl in the gastric contents was by giving a diet consisting of four meals a day: breakfast (8 a.m.) of oat porridge, eggs or white fish, milk or milky tea and toast; lunch (1 p.m.), cream soup, chicken,, rabbit, tripe or white fish and milk pudding; tea, toast and biscuits and milky tea; supper (6 p.m.) eggs or white fish, tea and toast. Judged by the nature of the stomach contents aspirated every hour, the four-meal diet was not emptied from the stomach as quickly as hourly or two hourly milk feeds, thus being given time to neutralise a considerable amount of the free HCl.

We also learnt, during this phase of the research, that not only physical but also psychological rest helped in the healing of ulcers, particularly duodenal ulcers. Hence the patients were given therapeutic doses of phenobarbitone night and morning. (By 'we' in the above paragraphs I mean Sister Clark and the nursing staff whose help was so willingly given, and myself, all of us under the stimulating direction of Professor Davidson.)

Stanley wasted no time in letting the pundits know the results of our work. He arranged to give a paper at a meeting of the Gastro-Enterological Club of the United Kingdom to be held in Cambridge early in 1938 and he insisted that I present the paper — my first experience of public speaking outside the lecture room. The membership of this club embraced many of the most senior physicians and surgeons in the country. My audience included Sir Arthur Hurst himself who chaired the meeting, sitting on the platform where I was talking and showing slides of our tables and graphs of the twenty-four-hour gastric acidity results. Sir Arthur was very deaf and held out an old-fashioned and intimidating ear trumpet towards me. Professor J. A. Ryle, developer of the Ryle's tube on which our work depended, Dr A. H. Doughtwaite, Sir Robert Hutchison, consulting physician to the London Hospital, and Professor Donald Hunter, also physician to the London Hospital and co-author with Sir Robert of my medical bible, *Clinical Methods*, Professor J. C. Spense, my friend from Newcastle days, and Sir David Wilkie, Professor of Surgery at the University of Edinburgh, were all among the audience. When I had finished, making it clear that neither Hurst nor Sippy diets met the claims made for them, Sir Arthur put down his ear trumpet and said to me in the loud voice of a deaf man, 'Do you mean to say, young fellow, that Dr Sippy and myself have been wrong for thirty years?' I had only time to say 'Yes, sir' when Stanley Davidson took over the handling of the brisk discussion which followed.

It is fitting to remark here, somewhat wryly, that fifty years later gastric acid output can be controlled and considerably reduced by the administration of what are called 'ulcer-healing' drugs which act 'as a result of their H_2-receptor blocking action. (BNF No. 7, 1984). So all the work done in dietary control of

WIND OF CHANCE

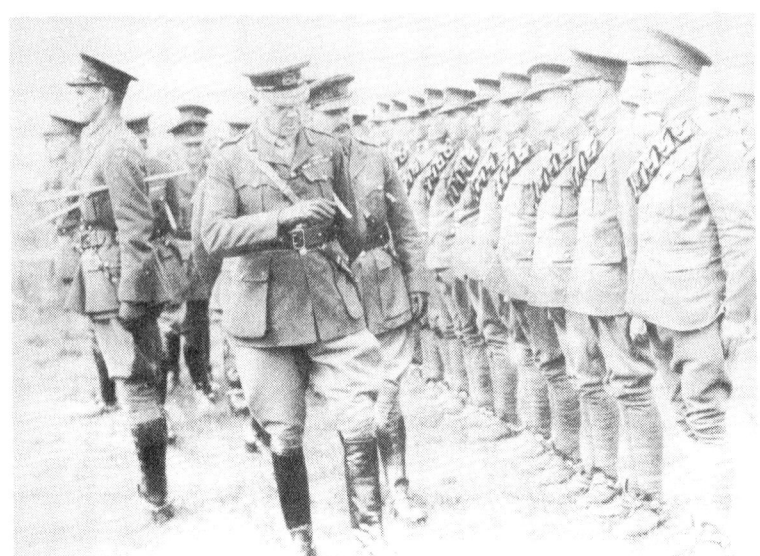

Territorial Royal Signals, the author on left.

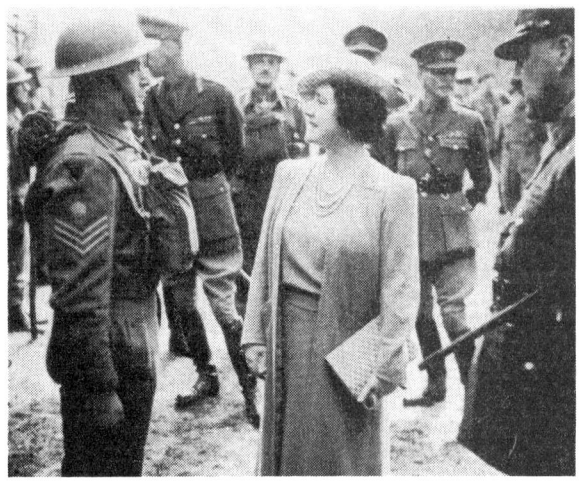

Brigadier Glyn Hughes on right, talking to Her Majesty Queen Elizabeth at Guards Armoured Division HQ, Wincanton, prior to landing at Normandy on D-Day plus 1. The author is behind Queen Elizabeth's hat.

gastric acidity is now at an end and arguments between Hurst and Sippy, Davidson and Nicol would not nowadays take place. However, the psychosomatic nature of duodenal ulcers and the physical trauma to the mucosa in gastric ulcer should still be borne in mind.

The professor was writing a book with Ian Anderson of Aberdeen called *A Textbook of Dietetics* which was published in 1940. In true Stanley style many of us in the Department of Medicine were called upon to help him and Ian to get the information accurate, go over drafts and proofs and to eliminate obscure sentences and meaningless phrases. Reg Passmore, who worked more than most people with Stanley on more than one book has written: 'Collaborating with Stanley was hard work, with many arguments but was always good fun.' Most of the time such hard work and argument was carried out in the evenings after a day's work and in Stanley's house outside Edinburgh, where he and Mrs Davidson were always most hospitable. I continued to imbibe knowledge and keenness for research from this stimulating environment until the beginning of the Second World War.

Military Service and the War Years

My first years of army service were spent in the Royal Corps of Signals. I joined the Territorial Army in 1933 when I was commissioned into the 51st (Highland) Divisional Signals, along with two friends of mine, also budding doctors, Alec Keith and Dyce Davidson. Our annual camps, lasting for two weeks in July, were very enjoyable and several of these were held near Leuchars aerodrome in Fife, countryside which I knew well as my Trail ancestors had been landowners in the area.

In 1939 our annual training took place at Aldershot and after that I went to Paris to stay with friends for a few days. On 28 August I felt I must get back to UK and once I'd arrived back at Newhaven I telephoned Fonthill Barracks, Aberdeen, to learn that we were to be mobilised the next day. I drove all 600 miles to Aberdeen in twelve hours.

At the beginning of October the Highland Division was moved to Aldershot to take the place of 1st Divisional Signals in Mons Barracks, who had already left for France. We carried out as much practical training as possible before transferring to Le

WIND OF CHANCE

Havre in the bitterly cold weather of January 1940. I was hoping to follow my two friends into the RAMC — Alec and Dyce had achieved this some months before but, for the time being, had to sit out the 'phoney war' in the area of Bethune, which was pleasant enough after the snow and ice finally melted.

One day in the Divisional HQ office I was approached by a man wearing the uniform of a major-general; he was not accompanied by anyone else. He was very tired and drawn and suddenly I realised it was the Duke of Windsor. He asked to see the Divisional Commander, General Fortune, so I showed him to General Fortune's office but I did not notice his departure. He had been given a liaison job but shortly afterwards was appointed Governor-General of the Bahamas.

I was unable to get into the RAMC then but that spring joined the 154 (Highland) Field Ambulance before the German invasion of Belgium and Holland in May.

German pressure increased eastwards towards the coast and it was clear we had to be evacuated. In June I found myself with other members of the Division embarked on the *Tynwald* at Cherbourg and sailing for Le Havre. On the night of 24 June the remaining officers and men of 154 (Highland) Field Ambulance were finally offered a passage towards Poole in a ninety-foot wooden diesel-engined boat under the command of a Royal Indian naval lieutenant who was based in Dorset. Fortunately he had plenty of fuel for as we set off he confessed that he had not swung his compass recently. Dawn broke but no land was yet in sight. A destroyer appeared and we were able to find out that we had just passed Portland Bill. We put about and finally reached Poole Quay. In the afternoon I was able to phone my family and reassure them of my safety.

In August confirmation of my deferred transfer to the RAMC arrived, through a letter from my bank.

> Dear Sir,
> We have now traced your transfer to the Royal Army Medical Corps. Details of this appeared in the *London Gazette* dated 30th July 1940, as follows:
> 'Captain B. M. Nicol, MB, from R signals TA to be Captain RAMC 18/5/40 with seniority 30/7/36'.
> We are arranging for the collection of arrears due to you.

PRACTISING AS A DOCTOR

The NCOs and other ranks were billeted in Bournemouth Town Hall but I was fortunate enough to be sent to one of the best hotels in town, the Palace Court.

The next day I unexpectedly met up with a cousin of mine, Douglas Jardine. That evening, somewhat reluctantly I must say, I joined him and Bill Watt, a New Zealand friend, to make up a group as the third man to partner three girls they had met that day for dinner. The following day Douglas took out his partner, Mary, but after a further two days I had managed to swop girls with him and Mary and I went off to dinner by ourselves. Her name was Dickinson and I learnt that her father had been mayor of Bournemouth the previous year. He was now deputy mayor and she acted as deputy mayoress as her mother had died earlier. I very soon had an inkling that she would become my wife. We had a wonderful evening but alas the next day I received marching orders for Dalbeattie where 154 Highland Field Ambulance was to be reassembled and reinforced.

During the next month I telephoned Mary whenever I could but often the lines between Scotland and England did not clear until around 2 a.m. One weekend I obtained leave to travel to Bournemouth and ask Mr Dickinson for his daughter's hand. He was very kind and to my surprise agreed immediately and said we should marry without delay. The thought crossed my mind that he wanted to get some decent rest at night without the telephone ringing but of course he was right that we should not procrastinate because there was a war on.

We were married in Bournemouth on 5 October 1940, with Bill Watt as best man, and Mary's friend Joan and two nieces and my sister Betty as bridesmaids. Mr Dickinson entertained our wedding party with some of our relatives from Aberdeen and London, to a hotel reception then Mary and I left for a brief honeymoon in Minehead.

Our first few months together were spent in Sussex before I was posted to Hawick in the Borders, and thence to Loch Fyne. I was stationed with the new 29 Independent Brigade Group on the merchant vessel *Stefan Battory,* with a Polish crew. During the time we were based at Loch Fyne the *Battory* was engaged in small-scale intelligence-gathering raids off Scandinavia and the Lofoten islands.

49

Mary spent this time in Bournemouth where she gave birth to our son, Christopher Bruce, known in the family as C., in November 1941.

My next job was as Deputy Assistant Director of Medical Services with the Guards Armoured Division, situated at Wincanton in Somerset. I remained with the Guards Armoured Division until 1945. I acted as medical officer for Divisional Headquarters and also undertook routine medical administration. Mary and Christopher and I were able to live together for some of this period. As the German bombing of the English cathedral cities progressed during 1942 (the Baedeker raids) we decided that Mary and C. would move north for safety and they went to live in Aberdeen, near my mother.

In February 1943 the Guards Armoured Division participated in the movement exercise 'Spartan' which took us right across southern England to East Anglia. The main Divisional HQ was at Cockley Cley in Norfolk. There, another officer and I found a lake overgrown with weed but well stocked with brown trout, and we realised we were both keen fishermen. Three of us then cleared a patch of weed from the bank and area of clear water and built a wooden platform whence we could cast a fly. For some reason the lake did not sport a boat. In this way we kept the mess well supplied with trout for dinner.

Unfortunately a severe outbreak of hepatitis occurred while we were there, affecting thirty officers. I was one of the earliest casualties and was sent to the Addenbrooke's Hospital, Cambridge. After about six weeks I was back on duty with strict instructions not to drink alcohol for a further three months.

After four months in East Anglia we moved on to Yorkshire for more intense battle practice. There I was promoted to the command of 19 (Guards) Light Field Ambulance. In March 1944 'my' unit had the honour of being visited by the King and Queen and the two princesses. We were undergoing an important phase of preparation for our move across the sea, which we knew could not be far off. I went to London to attend a course on the operation for crossing the Channel (Operation Overlord).

In June the time came to move to the concentration area in Sussex. The Division was part of the second wave to be transferred across to Normandy. My unit, with one hundred

PRACTISING AS A DOCTOR

vehicles, was ferried by a US-commanded Landing Ship Tank and landed west of Courcelles on 13 June.

While we were in Normandy my brother, padre to the 5th Battalion Black Watch, was also in the area and came to visit our Divisional HQ to see how we were getting on. After a few months in the region of Bayeux, the Division moved off on its first operation as a complete formation, Operation Goodwood, and I was soon involved in the evacuation of casualties of the anti-tank fire aimed at the village of Gagny. One afternoon I went to survey the ruins of Colombelles and Caen and encountered Norman Logie, surgeon and demonstrator to my anatomy class ten years earlier. He told me of the high proportion of fatalities suffered among casualties in another unit in the area. Two former co-students in my year in medicine, John Bain and Peter Ingram, had just operated on eighteen casualties, all of whom had died, but the conclusion was that they had been wrongly classified as Class IV and in fact they were all severely wounded and were Class III or even Class II.

Though 'Goodwood' must be counted as a costly failure we all learnt much of strategic and technical value from it. One day we had to deal with two unusual casualties, one Canadian and one from 43rd Division, who were not victims of war but curiosity. They had met in the cellar of a Norman farmhouse where they had found large casks of a yellowish fluid which they took to be cider and drank deeply of it. By chance they were found and when they were taken to the ADS both were comatose and suffering from acute alcohol poisoning, the fluid having been immature Calvados. The Canadian died almost immediately after admission but the British soldier was resuscitated by gastric lavage, coramine and artificial respiration. The Canadian had shown signs of shell-shock. The British troops suffered from this to some extent but it was far more prevalent among the US troops engaged in the battle for Cherbourg peninsula and they even had to set up 'exhaustion centres' to deal with it.

While we were still in Normandy I made a most important acquisition. For an exorbitant price I purchased two small pigs from a reluctant farmer. Until Christmas 1944 they travelled in a trailer behind the Dental Officer's truck. They were carefully tended by the dentist and quartermaster, fed on swill from the cookhouse and attained a very large size by the time they were slaughtered for Christmas 1944.

We moved on eastwards to take part in the liberation of Brussels and at the beginning of September had reached Douai. After the final ninety miles we arrived at the Belgian capital on the evening of 3 September but we had tremendous difficulty in passing through the crowds — it seemed the whole population was on the streets. I and my jeep driver Ives suddenly realised we were separated from the British troops. In the dark I came across one man who, from behind, looked familiar. Without regard for security I said to him, 'I am Colonel Nicol, commanding 19 (Guards) Light Field Ambulance. Do you know where 5 Guards Armoured Brigade HQ is?' He replied, 'I am Colonel Hill commanding 5 Battalion Coldstream Guards. Have you seen my bloody unit HQ anywhere?' I continued into downtown Brussels in my jeep to a street near the Bourse, where it became impossible to move. Ives and myself were lifted bodily from the jeep and marched straight into a bistro by some large gentlemen wearing white armbands, the Armee Blanche (Belgian Resistance). I was assured the jeep would not be stolen, which turned out to be true, and two bottles of champagne were opened and put on the counter 'pour le premier officer anglais qui a visité le quartier general de la compangie de la Resistance'. An hour later we were told by our hosts it was now known that our general's HQ was in the park in front of the Royal Palace. I was guided there by our new friends who, thanks to their insignia and arms, could make a way through the hysterical crowds and we found not only Divisional HQ and 5 Brigade HQ in the park but my own unit in a nearby school which had been found for it by Major Price, my second in command.

Brussels was illuminated during the whole of the night 3/4 September by the burning Palais de Justice, due to the Germans' attempt to destroy incriminating documents.

After Brussels we moved on to Hechtel which fell on 12 September but not before we had admitted more than 400 casualties, including thirty-five officers from the Division.

Our next objective, as part of Operation 'Market Garden', was to move in to the Netherlands via Eindhoven and Nijmegen to the Zuider Zee to cut off the eastward retreat of the German troops while allowing the Allies to out-flank the Siegfried Line at its northern end. The American airborne forces would be responsible for the Eindhoven Bridge and the area north to the Waal and the Meuse while the British would take care of the Lower Rhine beyond the Arnhem Bridge. The events of that month have been described in several books during the past three decades and will not be detailed here. We all had a rough time, the Light Field Ambulance dealing with large numbers of casualties though fortunately few fatalities, but we also had supply difficulties.

November saw us back in Belgium, preparing to clear the Reichswald and the west bank of the Rhine (Operation Veritable). At Christmas we ate our beautiful Norman pigs. After a muddy and freezing winter Operation Veritable got under way and, with the crossing of the Rhine at the end of March, the end of the war was in sight for us. Our subsequent advance towards the Elbe was severely impeded by the Germans, but we moved slowly eastwards and at the end of April we were in the region of Stade. One of our tasks was to help a local burgomeister against the Hitler Youth who were murdering his village population. One week later found us heading into town and on 6 May a group of officers, including myself, went to meet the surrendering German commander of the area, General Goltzach, to discuss the state of the roads and learn about the medical and other facilities available. We discovered that there was a total of around 25,000 officers and other ranks in and around Cuxhaven.

A POW camp was established near Cuxhaven airport for which 19 Light Field Ambulance took medical responsibility. Throughout the area of the Guards Armoured Division, the Nazi groups, including Hitler Youth, were sent to Sandbostel and Westertinke prison camps while the Wehrmacht officers and other ranks were sent to their homes to help with farming and get in the 1945 harvest, which would be of great importance to a defeated and starving country. Having dealt with them we were moved into the area around Sulingen west of the Weser and south of Bremen, where we found good billets.

Preparations were then started for the 'Farewell to Armour' parade, which took place on Rotenburg airfield on 9 June 1945. During the cleaning up and spit and polish period preceding the parade, the tanks, scout cars and artillery were all painted battleship grey with paint 'acquired' in Cuxhaven.

The few minutes between Brigadier Norman giving the command, 'Crews mount; start up', and the four columns of tanks disappearing over the ridge behind them, to be replaced by the seven columns of men marching as Foot Guards back over the ridge, was like a prolonged Armistice Day silence, full of memories of those never to be with us again. When the battalion had formed up, General Allen gave the command not heard since 1919, 'Guards Division Attention! God save the King.'

The Guards Armoured Division had advanced 700 miles from Bayeux to Cuxhaven, including the longest advance achieved in one day by any formation — 100 miles from Douai to Brussels.

Analysis of Casualties

The nature of the casualties and sick admitted to 19 (Guards) Light Field Ambulance from Normandy up to the end of the war in Germany is given in the table (see page 178). The figures reflect the heavy fighting encountered from Normandy to Nijmegan but also show that the battles across the Rhine towards Stade and Cuxhaven were as fierce as in the former period.

During the winter from November 1944 to March 1945 the sickness rate outstripped the battle casualties and battle accidents.

CHAPTER 4

Medical Service in India

September 1945 to January 1946

The powers that be in the Army Medical Services, Officers' Posting Department (AMD 1) had found out that I had pre-war experience in the Federated Malay States; they knew that I had served with 154 (H) Field Ambulance in Combined Operations Force 110 earlier in the war; they were aware that sea-borne invasion of Malaya on an unknown date was being planned by Admiral Louis Mountbatten following the successful conclusion of the Burma campaign in May 1945; and they knew they were short of experienced medical officers for this operation. Therefore it was logical to post me to Ceylon to participate in some way in this operation (known as 'Zipper' because it wasn't buttoned up). This logic resulted in my transfer to UK from 19 (Guards) Light Field Ambulance at the end of June 1945.

I was not given more than twenty-four hours to hand over to my successor who, by an extraordinary quirk of fate, was Lt.-Col. P. L. E. Wood, DSO, MBE, a regular RAMC officer — Phil Wood from my youth in Saxe Coburg Place.

It appeared, on the other hand, illogical to grant me two months' leave immediately I arrived in England in July 1945. However, I was issued with tropical kit at the RAMC depot and was sent to Edinburgh for three weeks to do a crash course in tropical medicine.

Eventually the news of the dropping of the atomic bombs on Hiroshima and Nagasaki on 6 and 9 August respectively came through. Obviously this new approach to warfare had upset the timing of Operation 'Zipper'. Nevertheless I was given instructions to report to Tilbury Docks to embark in the troopship *Johan de Wit* on 31 August 1945, destination probably Colombo.

Even so the ship did not sail until 3 September, full of troops to reinforce those in the Middle and Far East.

We were told that the *Johan de Wit* was the first troopship to pass through the Suez Canal since the end of the war in Europe and it was good to see the memorial at the north end — Défense du Canal de Suez 1914-1919 — quite undamaged after the desert campaign of early 1944. We sailed from Port Tewfik on 13 September 1945 after my third ship-borne passage through the Canal. It was with some surprise that I was disembarked in Bombay on 20 September having expected to go to Colombo. However, we were told that 'Zipper' was over and done with. In spite of the Japanese unconditional surrender on 14 August, Malaya, Singapore and the Dutch East Indies were still occupied by their troops. On 9 September a landing from Ceylon had been made at Klang, Port Swettenham, and other ports on the west coast of Malaya, concluding with a surrender ceremony in Singapore on 12 September 1945, thus clearing the Malacca Straits for traffic bound for points further east, including Hong Kong. The last time I had been in Port Swettenham and Klang was in April 1937.

The movement control officer in Bombay said that I was to take over command of the Combined Military Hospital (CMH) in Wellington, Nilgiri Hills, South India. I would travel to Madras the next day and report to the ADMS there. He was in the Indian Medical Services. (A combined military hospital is one which admits cases from both Indian and British armies serving in India.)

After two nights in the Taj Mahal Hotel in Bombay I found myself on a troop train *en route* to Madras. I was then taken to Spencer's Hotel in Madras where I spent twenty-four hours. I was introduced to the ADMS, Madras District, and to the secretary of the Madras Club where I was made an honorary member in view of my rank and posting in the Madras Medical District, which covered the political Presidency of Madras, Sir Arthur Hope being the Governor. In addition to the CMH Wellington I was responsible for the health of the Naval Staff College personnel in the military barracks in Ootacamund ('Ooty'), the hill station where Vivian Hartley (Leigh) had first appeared on stage in a children's pantomime at the age of three.

MEDICAL SERVICE IN INDIA

The reason I was urgently needed in the CMH Wellington, Operation 'Zipper' having been accomplished, was to take over from an elderly New Zealand medical officer who was suffering from cancer who wished to be retired and repatriated.

The Ooty barracks, for which I was responsible, where a small force had been maintained in former times, for the protection of Madras from the West, was very substantially built and old-fashioned. There was one English private practitioner who had a nursing home in Ooty and specialised in obstetrics and gynaecology.

Near the top of the Nilgiri Hills dwelt two indigenous tribes who appeared ethnically different from the Indians living at lower levels, the Todas and Budegas. They were bodily more hirsute than the Aryan peoples living below them. Their livelihood was derived from herding buffalo and selling the milk, butter and cheese in Ooty, Wellington and Coonoor.

Malaria-carrying mosquitoes did not exist at the altitude of the cantonment, 6,000 feet, but we treated many cases in the hospital; soldiers and naval staff who had come on leave to the hills and had been remiss in taking either mepacrine or quinine when posted on the coasts or plains of India or around Bangalore, where was Southern Command at that time, having been moved south from Poona during the war. A jungle warfare training centre was located at Gudaloor, on the road from Ooty to the city of Mysore, also in the Madras Presidency, where I was responsible for a hospital of 100 beds under canvas. One medical officer and two nursing sisters from CMH Wellington were seconded for monthly periods to this hospital and I visited it once a week. The drive was very interesting; across the grassy plateau of the Ooty downs; then down the steep ghat (mountain) road into the jungle, most of it bamboo; the occasional sight of sambur, tiger or elephant.

In view of the plentiful movement of military personnel to and fro between the non-malarial hilltops and the malarial jungles and plains, I decided that all hospital staff and patients admitted to hospital should routinely be given daily tablets of mepacrine. This was an unpopular innovation. Further I insisted that all patients on admission to hospital and all out-patients should have a blood film taken and examined for malaria parasites, whatever their presenting complaint or clinical features. In this way we correctly diagnosed and treated a number of cases of 'pyrexia of unknown origin' (PUO).

One day, while examining blood slides from Toda and Budega out-patients under the microscope, I observed, on three occasions, the red blood cells 'sickle', i.e. change shape from the normal circular state to that of a crescent or reaping hook. Neither I nor any other medical officer then on the staff of the hospital ever saw this 'sickling' in Indians of Aryan origin. Nor did we see any cases of sickle-cell disease among these primitive tribesmen. The microscopic changes in the red cells seen by us established only the the Todas and Budegas carried the heritable sickle-cell trait found in negroes in many parts of the world and among certain Mediterranean races. This heritable trait is due to an abnormality of haemoglobin. These two tribes were not negro or of Mediterranean origin. Or were they derived at some ancient time from, negro stock? I asked this question in a letter to the journal *Ecology of Food and Nutrition* in 1980.

The only other bit of work I initiated while commanding the CMH Wellington was concerned with the eradication of bubonic plague. There was a cordite factory a few miles from the centre of Wellington which had probably been functioning since the days of Warren Hastings's East India Company. Its employees were housed in very old wooden huts or 'lines'. The factory and its workers' lines were infested with rats which lived in deep burrows in the ground. In spite of frequent burning of the wooden buildings, pumping cyanide gas into the rat holes and the use of other rat poisons, the animals flourished. Our experience with dichlor-diphenyl-trichlorethane (DDT) as an insecticide in pressure-dusting the refugees returning westwards to Germany from across the Rhine in order to control the spread of lice and hence of typhus fever to Western Europe gave me an idea. DDT had not yet reached the Nilgiri hilltops but I managed to obtain a plentiful supply and some pressure-pumps from a commercial source in Madras. We pumped masses of DDT down the rat holes and, while the rats remained, their fleas which carried the germ causing plague, were killed. The prevalence of the disease among the coolies fell sharply, and the incidence became zero after six weeks.

Most of the officers and other staff were health graded B, i.e. unfit for active service because of such clinical features as flat feet or other locomotor complaints, poor eyesight, chronic chest troubles and so on. In addition to the British Matron (Queen Alexandra's Imperial Military Nursing Service) the staff was a mixture of both Indians and Europeans. The whole composition of the staff indicated how, in 1946, the IMS and British Medical Services were stretched to the limit on active service around the world, leaving the job of staffing combined military hospitals and such as that in Wellington mainly to the British Medical Services in India, most of the latter, moreover, being unfit for active service.

Due to the diverse origins of patients and staff, orderly room proceedings had to be conducted in one or other of six languages or vernaculars: Tamil, Telegu, Malayalam, Hindi, Urdu and English. Fortunately a young Tamil, who was employed as a *mali* (gardener) in the hospital compound, could translate the first three into English and *vice versa,* and Captain Oakley, the quartermaster who had soldiered all over India, could deal with Hindi and Urdu.

Even though the war in Burma was over the hospital was always full with convalescent, sick and accidentally injured patients. The bulk of the convalescent cases were sent up to us from the field hospitals complex at Jalahali near Bangalore which had been set up during the Burma campaign. As I have said, firm discipline was needed to keep malaria under control. Reasonably good control had been achieved in the armies fighting in Burma but on return to India the necessary discipline seemed to slip and relapses were often seen in casualties and convalescents. Other diseases which we had to treat in the CMH were dysentery, both bacillary and amoebic. A routine course of treatment for acute (vegetative) amoebiasis, lasting four weeks and based upon emetine, emetine bismuth iodide and stovarsol, had been drawn up by Brig. J. D. S. Cameron, consultant to Military HQ in Delhi. He was on the staff of the Edinburgh Royal Infirmary before and after the war. Sir Leonard Rogers, FRS, of the IMS, had introduced emetine in the treatment of amoebiasis in the 1920s.

Shortly after my arrival in Wellington a young lady from UK, who was in the FANYS (First Aid Nursing Yeomanry), a volunteer nursing service working with the army), was admitted to the CMH. She had spent three weeks in Bombay living in Green's Hotel and working in a military hospital there. She was to be posted to Wellington and had become feverish on the railway journey to Madras and then up to Coonoor. On arrival she had a hectic fever, extreme abdominal pain, an enlarged liver and vegetative forms of entamoeba histolytica in her faeces. It was apparent that she had an abscess in her liver and I decided to aspirate it the day after she was admitted. Fortunately that night the abscess perforated her diaphragm and she coughed up several ounces of the classical 'anchovy sauce' type of pus. After a full one month 'Cameron' course of treatment she made an uninterrupted recovery and was on duty within two months.

Venereal disease (both gonococcal and spirochaetal) was common in both officers and other ranks. A few cases of kala-azar in patients from the Bengal area and the general gamut of illnesses normally found in both temperate and tropical climates, e.g. bronchitis, pneumonia, cardio-vascular ailments and so on made up the overall list. Snake bite was a rare condition and the polyvalent antivenom developed by the Haffkin Institute covered all the local snake species.

Rabies was another threat to health in this area of India, the main reservoir being mongrel (pie) dogs and jackal. Suffice it to say here that it was in Wellington I learnt the unpleasantness, particularly when dealing with young children, of having to give fourteen daily prophylactic injections of vaccine to patients thought to have been exposed to infection. The only two occasions I have had the misfortune to see human beings dying of rabies was in Wellington Hospital. They were both sepoys.

My hospital duties and routine visits to Coimbatore and Gudaloor were not arduous, leaving many afternoons and evenings free for golf on the Wellington course, which was delightfully laid out on the side of a mountain. Where the tees were set back in tea bushes it was wise to send the caddie onto the tee to ensure that it was clear of the dangerous small snake called the krait. When I had to visit the barracks at Ooty I made time for more golf on the Ooty course which was situated on open down-like land, many of the holes being blind.

British India was a very conservative place before partition in 1947. For generations every officer, when a patient in hospital, was entitled to have either a large measure of spirits (whisky, rum or gin) or a bottle of beer per day, provided the MO in charge of his case allowed it. Regarding the spirit ration there was no difficulty — even if the gin had to be brought from Parry's in Madras or from Heyward's from Calcutta! The rum came from naval sources.

It was the supply of beer, apparently never questioned by my predecessors as Officers Commanding CMH Wellington, which surprised me. Many decades ago a brewery, the first in British India, had been opened at a small town called Murree, some distance from Rawalpindi on the North West Frontier. A contract had been established to provide the CMH Wellington with beer from this place, approximately 2,400 miles as the crow flies and at least 3,000 miles as the roads and railways meander. A consignment took six weeks to reach Wellington from Murree, most bottles broken en route, the contents of any whole ones being undrinkable. Meanwhile we bought excellent beer from the brewery recently established halfway between Wellington and Ootacamund, paying for it from PRI funds. This arrangement seemed ridiculously wasteful, and I took it up with the Major-General in charge of Administration (MGA) at Southern Command HQ, General Roy Boucher, an Edinburgh Academical. He looked into the matter and told me some weeks later that the situation was over one hundred years old and impossible to stop as more than sixty subcontractors were involved between Murree and Wellington. Very conservative, India, and the Indian Army!

On a visit to the ADMS in Madras I had the privilege of meeting one of Mary's aunts, Miss Gertrude Pearce. She was head of the social services department at the Buckingham and Carnatic Mills, a well-known textile complex north of the city. She was very musical and was the proud possessor of a very large collection of classical gramophone records which she played through an enormous horn, with bamboo needles. She had trained her head bearer to catalogue the records and operate the machine. All she had to do was to clap her hands and issue orders in Tamil and the music for which she had asked would issue through the horn.

Occasionally I met members of the staff of the Pasteur Research Institute at Coonoor which was then known on a worldwide basis as one of the leading research laboratories on the subject, thanks to pioneering work of Sir Robert McCarrison, FRS, IMS, into the causation of goitre and nutritional deficiency diseases and of his successor in 1935, Dr Wallace Aykroyd. Dr V. N. Patwardhan had

WIND OF CHANCE

taken over the Directorship from Aykroyd and Dr C. Copelan was his second in command.

Life was pleasant in the Nilgiri Hills, so I was making arrangements for Mary and C. to come out and join me there, and she was busy packing up to do so. I had a Territorial Army commission and had opted to defer my release from the army until such time as I found some congenial work to do. It had been taken for granted by Professor Stanley Davidson that I would rejoin his staff of the Department of Medicine at Edinburgh University after the war. However, he had told me that with luck he could pay me £600 per annum, only £100 more than I was getting six years earlier before the war. My yearly pay as a lieutenant-colonel in the RAMC was more than £1,300 at that stage and life in South India was pleasant. However, I did not know how long I could continue deferring my release from the British Army. So I took the path of least resistance and decided on the *status quo,* the hope being that Mary could come out soon to enjoy it with me, a hope which was never fulfilled due yet again to the outrageous intervention of Chance.

On 15 November 1945 I received a copy of a signal sent to me from Army Medical Services HQ in Delhi, which read as follows: 'British Service Medical Officers rank of Major and above *including* repeat *including* those who have deferred release will be repatriated immediately to United Kingdom by air transport.' The signal, which was sent to me direct from Delhi, bypassing Southern Command in Bangalore and District HQ in Madras, was accompanied by instructions to report to Erode, an RAF station halfway between Wellington and Madras, within forty-eight hours to be air-trooped to UK forthwith and to report to AMD 1, Hyde Park Gate, London, on arrival in UK. It did not tell me to whom I should hand over command of the CMH. Therefore I telephoned (it was possible to do so from Wellington) General Boucher, NGA, at Bangalore and the ADMS in Madras. Both were very surprised as they had not heard of any such order related to British MOs in India. The former immediately got in touch with the AM Services in Delhi who confirmed the signal to him and said they would have to comply but were checking with the War Office in UK. I cabled Mary to say I would be home for Christmas, left the CMH Wellington in the care of the quartermaster and the British service captain and reported to Erode as instructed.

It took fully six weeks to reach England, despite travelling by air, thanks to interminable delays spent in transit camps. We flew via Karachi, Lydda, Castel Benito (Libya) and Istres, and forty of us finally arrived back in England at RAF Waterbeach, Cambridgeshire.

Having spent the night at the University Arms Hotel in Cambridge, I took a train to London and reported to AMD 1, Hyde Park Gate. There I was sent to an office where sat an acquaintance from the early days of the war, Derrick Stevenson (he later became Secretary of the British Medical Association), whose first words to me were, 'What the hell are you doing here? You are supposed to be commanding the CMH, Wellington.' I placed the signal I had received from Delhi on his blotter while he produced a file and showed me a signal originated by himself eight weeks earlier which had exactly the same wording as my message except that, for the words in mine '*including* repeat *including* those who have deferred release', the original read '*excluding* repeat *excluding* those who have deferred release'. Stevenson's remarks about the High Command in India, politicians in UK, and various other subjects eventually died down and a startled look appeared on his face. 'How many others did you come back with? You are the first I have seen in this position.' When I told him about forty from only Southern Command in India he became very worried as to what the total from the whole of India and the rest of the world might be. Then he explained that Aneurin Bevan, the socialist Minister of Health in Attlee's government who was planning to, and did initiate, a National Health Service in 1946, was trying to flood the market with unemployed and senior medically qualified doctors in order to fully staff this child of the Welfare State and of the socialists and he, Stevenson, thought the unexpected postings of MOs back to the UK from the services might have something to do with Bevan's plan. I never heard if this was a true concept of the reason for my return to UK from India. Stevenson said all he could do immediately was to post me to the RAMC depot at Church Crookham, near Aldershot.

So ended my short, but informative, military service in India.

This posting to the depot was a piece of good fortune for me because it was commanded by none other than Brigadier Glyn

Hughes, my first ADMS in Guards Armoured Division and godfather to my son Christopher.

Hughie had constantly urged me, while I was at the depot, to apply for a regular commission in the RAMC. I was uncertain about doing so, as a permanent life in army surroundings did not then appeal to me. I realised that I was far out of date with the practice of medicine, having spent the previous seven years in the army either as a signals officer or doing rough and ready casualty surgery in the forward areas during the war in Europe 1944-45. However, in the end I took the easy way out and sent in my application. The War Office took some time before turning me down. Then a fellow officer in the depot whose short service commission was about to terminate, and I gave some thought to joining the Colonial Medical Service. Very soon neither of us would have jobs, we had families to support and neither of us wanted to join Bevan's National Health Service. So we wrote to the Colonial Office, received forms to record our *curricula vitae* and within a week we were both asked to report to an Interview Board in Victoria Street, London. The interview was comprehensive. Within another week we had both been accepted as medical officers in the Colonial Medical Service. The form we had to complete for the Board's information gave an option of three colonies in order of preference. I put the Federal Malay States first, because I had been there before the war and had liked the approach of the Colonial Service doctors I had met in Singapore and Penang; Hong Kong second for the same reasons, although realising it had less scope; and the South West Pacific third, because I had never been there. The Board explained carefully that the medical officers who had survived the Japanese occupation of the FMS and Hong Kong had already been rehabilitated and returned to duty and that their establishments of MOs already had been filled. A policy of recruiting MOs for the S.W. Pacific from New Zealand and Australia had been implemented since the war's end. But how would I like to be posted to Nigeria, and up-and-coming West African territory? I had hardly ever heard of Nigeria. The chairman of the Board said that it was the most populous country south of the Sahara and that its establishment of MOs, including physicians and surgeons, was expanding as fast as the Colonial Office could finance the posts, that salaries were good (which

MEDICAL SERVICE IN INDIA

indeed they were), that home leave was earned at the rate of a week a month during a maximum tour of eighteen months, and that the climate in the hinterland plateau was good. Nothing was said about the coastal climate. At this point in his description many people would think I should have smelt a rat. However, I did not, and accepted the offer and can honestly say that I never, never regretted the decision.

When I returned to the depot that evening I found a patronising memorandum from AMD 1 saying that the War Office had changed its mind and now offered me a permanent commission from 1 January 1947 with the rank of major. I derived some pleasure in being able to tell the Army Medical Services that their memorandum had reached me a day too late. This touch-and-go timing was the most important event which ever happened, or was to happen, in changing the course of my life and my future professional work and interests.

I had been appointed to the Colonial Medical Service early in October and was given one month's leave (paid) from the Army Medical Service, and a gratuity of £80 before being allowed to resign my Territorial Army commission which I had assumed in 1933. Between that year and 1946 I had become eligible for the Territorial Decoration, the qualifications being twenty years' service without detected crime, war service counting double. This decoration became due just before I departed the RAMC depot in October 1946. I left Fleet and the army happily.

CHAPTER 5

Early Service in Nigeria

Having acquired the equipment and clothing recommended by the Colonial Office I sailed from Glasgow on 23 November 1946 leaving Mary and C. behind. The ship was filled with colonial civil servants who had been demobilised from the forces, with others who were returning from post-war leave, and also with new recruits to the Colonial Service, like myself. In this last category were young administrative officers (cadets) fresh from universities who had neither been in the army nor in Africa before, as well as older men such as me who did not know Africa but who were experienced specialists of one form or another. In my cabin, which in peace time would have provided two beds, were six large men sleeping on two sets of three shelf-like bunks, one of them a field gunner with service in Burma who, pre-war, had been a senior district officer in the British Cameroons, another the head postmaster for Northern Nigeria returning from post-war home leave. He had worked in Nigeria throughout the war as his job was regarded as a 'reserved occupation'. These two were about my age, at that time nearly thirty-four years. They told horrific tales about their previous service in Nigeria. The other three in the cabin were first-time out administrative cadets. The ship off-loaded a few personnel in Bathurst in the Gambia, more at Freetown in Sierra Leone, even more at Sekondi-Takoradi for the Gold Coast, but most of the passengers continued to Lagos, Nigeria.

Nigeria is an enormous country of 373,000 square miles, four times the area of the United Kingdom, with a population at the time of 31.5 million, 80 per cent of whom lived in small towns of less than 1,000 persons, villages, hamlets or separate houses. It was the most populous country in Africa divided administratively into three regions: Northern, with administration headquarters in

EARLY SERVICE IN NIGERIA

Kaduna; Eastern, with the administration based on Enugu; and Western, administered from Ibadan.

I was met in Lagos on 15 December 1947 by the Assistant Director of Medical Services (ADMS) Carl Wilson, who kindly put me up in his house in Ikoyi, then the European residential area of Lagos. He was a graduate of the old-fashioned Aberdeen medical school, i.e. the school which depended for professors upon private consultants in medicine, surgery and obstetrics, before the advent of Stanley Davidson, James Learmonth and Dougald Baird. He knew both the Nicol and Trail sides of my family. From him I learnt that the Medical Services in Nigeria were run on a federal (i.e. territorial-wide) basis, the Director of Medical Services (DMS) being Dr John Walker, known to everyone as Joey Walker; the Deputy Director (DDMS) was Dr Alexander (Sandy) Rae and he himself was number three in hierarchy as ADMS. All three Scotsmen were based in Medical Headquarters, the Marina Lagos, in a building facing the Lagoon. The town was founded in the fifteenth century by the Portuguese, on the island they called Lagos after the Algarve town of the same name in Portugal meaning 'lake'. From Lagos Dr Walker did a considerable amount of touring, trying to visit each medical officer at least once in his eighteen months of duty. Dr Rae was responsible at HQ for the technical aspects of the medical service and Dr Wilson for administration. The DMS was responsible to the Chief Medical Officer in the Colonial Office. Dr Wilson's duties included the ordering and distribution of medical stores throughout the country from the medical stores at Yaba on the mainland.

Politically the Governor of Nigeria was responsible to the Colonial Office for the Colony of Lagos, a small area of the town of Lagos on Ikoyi Island (the town of Lagos on Ikoyi Island was connected with the mainland and Colony by only one bridge, Carter Bridge); for the three regions, Northern, Western and Eastern, forming the Protectorate of Nigeria; and for the Trust Territory on the eastern border of the Protectorate known as the British Cameroons, north and south. The Governor, with his HQ and Federal Secretariat in Lagos, delegated responsibility to a Chief Commissioner for each region. The regions were composed of Provinces under the control of Residents. The medical areas were geographically designed to cover as many districts of a Province including one or more political divisions. Medical officers were directly responsible to the DMS Lagos administratively, but sent copies of their quarterly reports to the Provincial Resident and the SDO or DO in whose area they worked. Lord Lugard, I was told, had introduced a system of administration known as Indirect Rule, which supported and tried to improve the long-established dynastic authority of native chieftains by reducing cruelty and corruption. By and large the chiefs and their traditional responsibilities were not curtailed. Local laws and customs were overseen in the tribally established courts, presided over by the 'Alkali' or his pagan (i.e. non-Muslim) equivalent. The same principles applied in the Western and Eastern regions, where long-established chiefs had ruled for generations but where early missionaries had established a degree of Christianity, through such dedicated people as Mary Slessor (Church of Scotland) in the East and American missions in the West. In all regions a number of missions were run by the Roman Catholic Church.

Thus a two-tier system of government had been set up, the traditional legal and administrative organisation known as the Native Authorities (NAS) and the Government Administration and Judiciary System based on British principles.

In the Western Section the lingua franca is 'Yoruba', in the East 'Ibo' and in the Northern Region 'Hausa' and 'Fulani'. However, hundreds of languages specific to individual tribes were spoken throughout the whole country. British DOs were expected to learn one or other lingua franca, depending upon the region to which they were posted. Officers of the other services were paid a 'language allowance' if they passed the set examinations, which were of two standards, normal and higher level, but it was not obligatory for them to do so. During my three days in Lagos I met a new recruit to the medical service, Leonard Bruce-Chwatt, a Polish citizen by birth who was then engaged in trying to control the malaria endemic on the Apapa, or west side of the Lagos Lagoon, by constructing a drainage system to eliminate the local swamps. He was eventually to become a world authority on the control and treatment of malaria through his service in Nigeria, with the World Health Organisation and at the Wellcome Research Foundation.

Dr Wilson very kindly 'gave' me his number two houseboy, an Ibo called Chikizi, to be my 'number one' houseboy. Chikizi, who had been brought up in an RC mission near Port Harcourt, enrolled a 'Christian' Ibo friend of his as my first cook-boy, Bernard. He also enlisted, on his own initiative but to be housed and fed by me, a 'small boy' called Azuzu, a close relative.

I had been posted as MO to the Bida Medical Area in the southern part of the Northern Region, where the hospital was administered and staffed by the Bida Native Authority (NA) under the Emir of Bida, or Etsu Nupe in his own tribal language. I was to take over from Dr Oswald Macnamara.

Bida was one of two medical postings in Niger Province, at 28,000 square miles in extent only the fourth largest province in Northern Nigeria, and about 30 per cent of the area of the United Kingdom. The headquarters of the province was in Minna where the Residency and government offices were established.

Dr Macnamara, from whom I was taking over, told me much more about the extent of my responsibilities as MO Bida than had been vouchsafed by the ADMS, Carl Wilson. My medical 'parish', the western part of Niger Province, was approximately 19,000 square miles (one-fifth the area of the United Kingdom) in which lived 473,000 people, an overall density of twenty-five persons per square mile. My next door medical colleague was based in Minna, 150 miles away from Bida by the shortest road. This road had a corrugated red laterite surface throughout. His area was comparatively small by Northern Nigerian standards, 9,600 square miles, or one-tenth the area of UK with a population of 243,000, also twenty-five persons per square mile.

Dr Bill Berry tells us in his book, *Before the Winds of Change*, that when he joined the Colonial Medical Service in Nyasaland in 1936, the DMS had nine medical officers to serve in a country only 40 per cent the size of the United Kingdom, with a population of approximately two million or about 22,000 persons being the responsibility of one MO at an overall population density of fifty-three per square mile. These figures should be compared with the situation in Niger Province, Northern Nigeria, given above.

The MO Bida was responsible for the public health in the following native authorities: Bida Emirate, the headquarters of the Nupe kingdom presided over by the Emir of Bida or Etsu

Nupe as he was known in his own language, HQ in Bida; the Agaie Emirate, HQ 180 miles north of Bida Town; The Chiefdom and Council of Zuru, seventy miles north of Kontagora, nearly 250 miles from Bida.

These different NAs were responsible for the building and staffing of one hospital in Bida town of 200 beds, 120 for men and eighty for women and children.

Some of the staff were southerners who had been trained in nursing in Lagos, Ibadan (Western Region) or Enugu (Eastern Region). Training was given in Bida to local Nupe staff who made good nursing orderlies and midwives. To deal with the outlying areas fifteen dispensaries had been built and staffed by the different NAs close to major villages. In even more remote areas central to small groups of hamlets, nineteen dressing stations had been established. The dispensaries were staffed by one or two qualified dispensary attendants and one midwife trained either in Bida or in Kaduna General Hospital. The dressing stations were staffed by one or two 'dressers', who had had a short course on nursing in Bida or Kaduna hospitals. All dispensary attendants and dressers were trained to vaccinate against smallpox and give simple medicines on their own responsibility. The most distant of the dressing stations from Bida was fifty miles north of Zuru on the river Ka, 320 miles by motor vehicle, bicycle and horse from Bida town. I decided it would be one of my first targets when I started touring.

Dr Macnamara said he had been kept busy in the hospital dealing with a variety of tropical diseases as well as the diseases commonly found in countries of the climatically temperate regions of the world — bronchitis, pneumonia, tuberculosis, VD, gastro-enteritis, and so on. He had observed that the prevalence of cardio-vascular disturbances and nephritis was low. He had written a memorandum to the DMS on the subject of malnutrition as evidenced by poor growth rate in children and features of vitamin B deficiency of which he gave me a copy. He told me how to indent for medical supplies and explained that he had visited all the fifteen dispensaries during his eighteen months tour but only five of the dressing stations. He also pointed out that the quality of medical service varied from one dispensary or dressing station to another not so much due to the competence of the staff concerned but depending upon the interest taken in the health of the people by the Native Administration responsible. The varying interests of the administrative district officers and of the provincial Resident were also of great importance because they could interfere with one's plans in respect of the NAs. I noted this observation of his at the time but did not become fully aware of its fundamental importance until later in my tour in Niger Province and elsewhere in the Colonial Medical Service in Nigeria, and much later in its even wider implications at international level when I became involved with the United Nations and certain of its specialised agencies in questions concerning famines and food production in relation to community health and nutrition.

A further comparison between the respective colonial medical services in Northern Nigeria and Nyasaland seems to me worth noting. In 1936-43 Bill Berry had to spend a great deal of time on paper work and bureaucracy, but we in Nigeria were not unduly side-tracked from the practice of medicine by office work. In Bida I had two excellent clerks, of southern origin, one Ibo from the Eastern Region and one Yoruba from the Western Region, who dealt with all routine work needed. Emergency equipment would take about three weeks to arrive in Bida. But there are exceptions to everything. After I had been in Bida for about six weeks a very fine new operating table was delivered to the hospital, with hydraulic pumps for adjusting its height, angle of tilt and such like improvements on the rather elderly simple table I had inherited. It was addressed to the MO Bida, c/o Native Administration, Bida Emirate. No one could tell who had indented for it and the SDO told me not to use it until more information was available. In view of the turnover of staff not only in the District office and the Native Authority but in the hospital as well, it took three weeks to find out that it had been ordered by Dr Macnamara's predecessor's predecessor. A special order had been made to England for it and the NA had already paid for it. Then, and only then, was I allowed to assemble it and use it with some delight.

The MO of any Northern Region medical area was responsible not only for the care of out-patients and patients being treated in hospitals, dispensaries and dressing stations, he was also the medical officer of health and thus in charge of the native authorities' sanitary inspectors and orderlies. This implied supervision of water supplies, disposal of excreta, control of mosquito breeding and, for good measure, attempts to prevent the transmission of diseases such as schistosomiasis (bilharzia) or ankylostomiasis (hookworm disease) through prevention of the respective larvae penetrating the human skin from pools of water or damp ground, particularly around wells. Another duty was to ensure the sanitation of the slaughter-slabs where cattle were killed according to Muslim ritual. The sanitary inspectors and their teams also vaccinated against smallpox.

Although the administrative headquarters of Niger Province was in Minna for purposes of geography and communications, the major trading centre was Bida, at 25,000 population by far the largest and most important town in the province. Yet the European population of Minna was around thirty (government officials, railway staff, missionaries, merchants and their families). In Bida the equivalent figure when I arrived at the end of 1946 was nine — an SDO and his wife, an ADO, a PWD officer, an education officer, a representative of John Holt's trading firm and his wife, and myself. An English Church Missionary Society (CMS) pastor had a small mission station on the north-east of Bida town, just outside the old walls. He held Anglican services every Sunday morning and taught the local people to grow vegetables. He had trouble with hyenas which were liable to attack his flocks of sheep if they were not properly housed at nights.

Dr Macnamara handed over to me in two days and caught a train from Zunguru to Lagos, hoping to reach there for Christmas. I spent my first Christmas in Nigeria for dinner with the lady education officer, Joan Foster, and the PWD engineer, Bill Dempster. They introduced me to the others on the station during pre-dinner drinks parties held between Christmas and the New Year 1946-47.

After the Christmas and New Year festivities were over the SDO was asked by Etsu Nupe to introduce 'his' new doctor to him. On this first visit to the Etsu's palace I was impressed by the gloom and coolness inside the entrance hall and by the decorated china plates embedded in the vaulted roofs of the public rooms, where sat his bodyguard, courtiers and people awaiting an audience with the King of the Nupe empire. Until conquered by the Fulani, the Nupe had been a warlike people, raiding southwards into Yorubaland and selling slaves down the Niger River. In 1947 the Etsu was Mallam Mohanadu Ndayako, Etsu Nupe and Emir

EARLY SERVICE IN NIGERIA

of Bida. He was an imposing looking middle-aged, sturdy man dressed in a white riga (robe) and turban who greeted me very graciously in Hausa, the SDO acting as interpreter. He said that I would be medically responsible for his own person and that of the male members of his family. A young boy of about five years, currently his favourite son, was called for and shook hands with me very politely, and then ran away suffering from shyness. I said I was expecting my own five-year-old son and my wife to join me as soon as transport from UK was available. He said this was good and that the two boys must become friends. We shook hands and the interview was over. The SDO said, when we returned to the office, that the Etsu was being merely polite when he had talked about friendship between his son and mine. However, not only our sons but the Etsu and myself became good friends and he added the medical care of his wives and concubines to my duties in his palace, the one proviso being that when I entered the harem area I should be accompanied by my wife, Mary. She and I found this an interesting experience. The one person at court to whom I was never introduced nor saw was the Etsu's mother, reportedly a strong power behind the throne.

After Mary and C. arrived around the middle of March 1947 the Etsu developed a habit of asking himself to tea in our bungalow and, while he and I talked shop about the medical and public health aspects of his 'kingdom', the five-year-olds played outside under the care of one of the bodyguards. For them language did not seem to be a problem, but all my own conversations had to be carried out through an interpreter.

Anticipating events a little, I had selected Mallam Abubakar Zukogi-Bida, a trained hospital assistant and senior orderly, to help me with the food consumption surveys which I considered must be carried out in order to have a proper background to the various diseases and physical conditions I was being called upon to treat in the hospital and dispensaries. (The term 'Mallam' implies literacy and a grounding in the practices of Islam, in general terms a literate person.) Mallam Abubakar was a nephew of one of the Etsu's 'educated', i.e. literate councillors, Mallam Abuja, Makaman Bida, who had been headmaster of the Bida Middle School, the major school in Niger Province. Mallam Abubakar was a very intelligent and hardworking man who stayed with me in various capacities throughout my service in Nigeria (excluding only my postings to Warri and Lagos). Thus he translated from my English into Nupe or Hausa, whichever the Etsu felt like speaking and vice-versa. At these tea parties the Etsu drank tea while his son consumed large quantities of fruit juice. Christopher also drank fruit juice and always watched, wide-eyed, as the 'king' put more and more lumps of sugar into his teacup, until one lump broke the surface. Only then did he drink his tea and the two youngsters went out into the garden to play with C.'s first present from the Etsu, a tethered 'crown-bird' or crested crane, *Balearica pavonina*.

The Etsu told me that, for the time being, the prisoners in gaol were not giving any trouble but they sometimes complained about their rations being inadequate for the amount of work they were expected to do. Would I please look into the question and report to him. He also said, with some pride, that since he had become Emir in 1936 the Middle School had been moved from near the banks of the Lanzu stream, which runs through the town, to higher ground on the south-west, with the school dormitory nearby and close to the hospital. The middle school was a boarding establishment receiving children from neighbouring emirates and tribal areas. Since the move of the school from the stream banks the incidence of 'lunacy' among the pupils had fallen sharply. This interested me because Dr Macnamara had not mentioned it when handing over and I had seen that a number of adolescents and young men were confined in the 'lunatic asylum', euphemistically called as it was built as a series of lions' dens at a zoo, each with a front area open to the fresh air and sun but securely barred and an enclosed covered area behind for seclusion and sleep. I wondered if the schoolboys were being pushed too hard with their education and developing schizophrenia but Mallam Bida assured me this was not so — he had encountered such schizophrenic cases when he himself was a schoolboy at the famous secondary school run in Katsina, where most of the successful Northern Nigerians who became chief councillors to illiterate though shrewd emirs, or obtained work as colonial government servants, had been taught.

I finally tracked down the cause of the madness to 'sleeping sickness' (Trypanosomiasis), the infection being carried by the tsetse fly *glossina palpales* which lives and multiplies along shady stream banks and causes a form of brain disturbance, the clinical features of which are intermittent fever, and lethargy, interspersed with occasional attacks of mania. The lymph glands in the neck are often enlarged and the diagnosis can be made by finding the trypanosome in these glands. As both the 'lunatic asylum' and the prison were still beside the Lanzu and both prisoners and lunatics alike were liable to infestation, and probably reinfestation if in the same area for some months or years, I had to recommend that they be moved elsewhere to healthier terrain as had been done with the Middle School.

Etsu Nupe also forecast during one of our tea-parties that when the DMS from Lagos next visited me in Bida he would ask why the 'borrow-pits', which I had noticed around the town, had not been filled in since his last visit some eighteen months ago. 'Every time he comes he asks this question, but he does not understand the difficulties and man-hours and transport involved. Of course you understand the situation and please explain to him why we have not been able to do anything about them since his last visit. The first time he noticed them was well before the war started but he never forgets. I know that you order the sanitary inspectors to spray the water in them daily with oil to keep down the mosquitoes.' The rains had not broken when he told me this cautionary tale and I had not yet seen the deep water which drained into the vast, steep-sided craters which had resulted from the digging of huge quantities of mud with which to build the walls of the town and large palaces for the three main branches of the royal Nupe families from which the Etsu was appointed, not to speak of the walls of the round huts for the general population. The Nupe were excellent thatchers, working outwards in a circular fashion from a central apex. They could also thatch horizontally, from ridge poles, my bungalow being an example.

Work in the Bida Hospital

I had been asked to look into the state of the prison diet and had decided I should also investigate the Middle School diet and that provided by the hospital for 'pauper patients', i.e. patients who did not have relations or friends from Bida to bring them all their food from outside sources. But before starting that work I decided to spend at least a month working full time in the Bida Hospital and in the town, to gain some knowledge of the West African clinical and public health scene.

A day in the hospital started at 7 a.m. with out-patients. The presenting symptoms varied from 'fever', coughs, general aches and pains, belly-ache, skin rashes, loss of weight and energy, and swollen bellies; injuries caused by falls, bicycle accidents or reputed snake bites. Inguinal hernias in men were very frequent, also 'elephantiasis', caused by infestation with one of the filaria worms carried by mosquitoes, *Filaria or Wuchereria Bancrofti*; the filaria worms blocked the lymphatic system in the lower extremities thus causing swelling of the legs and scrotum in men and labia in women, combined with thickening of the skin. As in Europe or elsewhere in the world femoral hernias were more frequent in women than in men. I had not expected the women to come to hospital as readily as they did. Here the locals were served by both witch doctors and native medical men. It is necessary to clarify the difference between the witch doctor and the native medicine man. The first is usually an evil-doer practising 'ju-ju', or psychology; the latter is a local medical general practitioner using his own armament of medicines usually obtained from local plants, and is able to set fractures, dress wounds, incise abscesses like a GP in other countries. Etsu Nupe introduced me to his native medicine and compared it with mine. Witch doctors did not exist in Niger Province and few were found in Northern Nigeria, but the native medicine man did a lot of good, with traditional though limited knowledge.

From the rabble of out-patients, careful selection had to be made before admission because beds were limited in number, emergency cases taking top priority were high (120° F+) fevers and pyrexias of unknown origin (PUO). They were admitted to and isolated in the infectious diseases ward which was separate from the rest of the hospital. Second priority were acute undiagnosed abdominal conditions, most of which were found to be acute gall bladder inflammation or gall-stones, occasionally an obstructed or strangulated hernia, quite often amoebic hepatitis with or without abscess formation. Third priority were patients suffering from genito-urinary troubles such as acute retention of urine due to strictures of the urethra (seldom due to enlarged prostate lands, and this I attributed to the sexual activity of these men into comparatively old age). Of course we also had the occasional complicated labour which had been allowed to continue too long at home by the completely unqualified handiwives who practised midwifery unofficially in the town and surrounding villages. Most of these poor women, often teenage girls of fifteen years and upwards, had been in labour so long there was little I could do to treat post-partum haemorrhage in the absence of plentiful tranfusion fluids (blood and plasma) to which I had become accustomed during the war. However, an occasionally successful Caesarian section coupled with good nursing seemed to please the families and my two well-trained midwives on the hospital staff. I found the general standard of nursing to be higher than I expected. Two senior nurses in particular were quite competent anaesthetists using 'rag and bottle' ether — we did not have any Boyle's machines so gas and oxygen was out of the question. Therefore I decided it was justifiable to try and regain my surgical touch, much blunted by the war and service in India.

It should be made clear at this point that, although Muslims and non-Muslims alike were polygamous, very few of the simple peasant farmers could afford more than one wife and that a large family of at least five or six children, if not more, was hoped for by those people. They knew only too well that up to half of their live-born children would die before the age of five and it was necessary to have a surplus to ensure the continuation of the family on their own land and took look after them in their old age. A childless couple were to be pitied.

Of course I had 'acute abdomens' to do all the time I was in the Bida area and even some in dispensaries when on tour. These varied from removal of gall bladders, incisions and drainage of amoebic abscesses, urethral dilations to breakdown strictures caused by gonorrhoea, removal of bladder stones, some of which were enormous, and bowel reactions and repair in some cases of strangulated hernia. Acute and chronic appendicitis and diverticulosis were noticeable on account of their complete absence. This may be due to the bulky diets eaten, containing much fibre. Such major surgery could not be done in the hospital when I was on tour around my large district visiting dispensaries and dressing stations and many people who could have been saved must have died. The hospital staff, while excellent at dealing with minor illnesses and capable of performing minor definitive surgery and first aid, were philosophic about the situation. As my senior nurse, an Ibo from Calabar in the Eastern Region and a Christian, often told me, 'You cannot be in two places on this earth or in Niger Province at the same time, thank God.'

Regarding medical cases, those admitted to the infectious diseases ward with PUO were diagnosed generally sooner than later by their developing symptomatology. Possibly a smallpox rash developed in which case they were isolated in a few huts which were located just outside the town walls far from the nearest compound, where they were nursed by two dedicated men who had had the disease some years before. The sanitary inspectors then vaccinated or revaccinated all traceable family and other contacts. Respiratory diseases such as bronchitis and lobar pneumonia were nursed in the hospital ward, as were patients with severe malaria or amoebiasis for which specific treatment was available. Patients suffering from tuberculosis were isolated in a separate ward, unfortunately often full and treated symptomatically as neither isoniazid nor streptomycin had yet reached Nigeria. As many out-patients as possible were sent home with simple medicines for coughs, chalk and opium mixture for diarrhoea which did not appear to be bacillary dysentery, but may well have been as the local population had acquired a partial immunity to many diseases of infectious origin, including leprosy. Fortunately, while I was MO Bida I did not encounter any of the serious and deadly epidemics of measles or cerebro-spinal meningitis (CBM), about which we had all been warned in tropical medicine courses. They occurred more often in the more northerly provinces during the dry season.

When I was on tour the out-patient department continued to function under the supervision of the senior nurse. 'Tropical' ulcers on the lower third of the leg, attended for their routine dressings, accidents and injuries were given first aid, yaws and syphilis were treated by intramuscular injection of organic arsenicals and cases of gonorrhoea with sulphonamides. Fortunately the Bida gonococci were not resistant to sulphathiazole at this point in time as a result of under-dosage, as were the gonococci acquired by United States forces in Europe, who had developed the bad and unauthorised habit of eating the four tablets supplied in their first field dressings, hopefully as a prophylactic, instead of crumbling them to powder and putting it in their wounds before applying the dressing.

EARLY SERVICE IN NIGERIA

The ante-natal, post-natal and follow-up maternity clinic started by Dr Macnamara continued to be held at 3 p.m. once a week during my absence from the station. The senior midwife was meticulous about weighing the babies from birth onwards up to the age of two years. The weighing was done on a proper yard-arm balance and I found that the technique had been taught to the midwives and other nurses very satisfactorily.

The Nupe nursing orderly responsible for our hospital medical store and for issuing stores to the out-patient department and wards was scrupulously honest and we had no trouble with missing drugs or dressings. In fact I was very impressed by the previous training and competence of the staff at Bida, and my first experience of a hospital in the wilds of Nigeria, particularly as it happened in the immediate post-war period. The Colonial Medical Service in Nigeria appeared to have survived the war very well.

Bush Touring — First Time Around the Area

Having become acquainted with the Bida Hospital the next thing to do was to make a preliminary tour of my medical area. A major snag was the post-war lack of transport, which affected the personnel of all departments. Therefore Joan Foster and I decided that it would be mutually advantageous to share a three-ton lorry provided by the Bida NA and to share the cost of hiring it between our two departmental budgets. We both sat in the cab with the driver and our 'loads' (touring equipment including personal bedding, cooking stoves, and medical and educational materials) were in the body of the lorry. When we reached our destination she would occupy the rest house and Chikizi would put up my Houndsfelt bed, with the mosquito net, outdoors.

My first tour with Joan Foster (now Mrs Russell and still a good friend forty years later on) took us first to Kontagora, so that for the first time I could meet the head of the second biggest emirate in my district, that of Kontagora, established in the early eighteenth century by Fulani from Sokoto. Sarkin Sudan, Umaru Maiduru was the Emir of Kontagora when I first went there on this tour. Afterwards I visited dispensaries further north in the Zuru chiefdom. These pagan tribes had never been conquered by the Fulani. On the way to Kontagora I visited dispensaries at Lemu and at Zunguru, both the responsibility of the chieftain of Wushishi, sixty miles from Bida, and at Tegina, twenty miles north of Zunguru. The large dispensary in Kontagora town, sixty miles west of Tegina, where Mallam Isa Likata was the well-known attendant, was followed by a visit to the dispensary at Dabai, sixty-five miles north of Kontagora, and a dispensary at Zuru, thirty miles north of Babai — in all an outward journey of 235 miles to see six dispensaries. The nursing staff and midwives seemed to know their jobs and have reasonably good attendances at their out-patient sessions. I was given lists of drugs and dressings which had been exhausted or were in short supply so that I could indent for more medical stores. This tour took place in the first half of February 1947, when I felt I was established in Bida Hospital.

We decided to make a diversion on the homeward journey to visit a dressing station and elementary schools at Ibeto on the Kontagora-Yelwa road and at Auna near the Niger river south of Yelwa, close to the Bussa rapids where Mungo Park had been drowned in 1806 during his trip down the Niger from Timbuktu. Halfway between Ibato and Auna, on the track which was only open to cars and lorries during the dry season, an American mission was established and run by a preacher and his wife. They had a two-month-old baby which had been born in Kaduna Nursing Home. The child appeared healthy and was being breast-fed satisfactorily by its mother. A well-established orchard of grapefruit, guavas, limes and lemons showed that the mission had been established for many years. The pastor said that he did not have many converts to Christianity from the local Kamberri pagan tribe, who had been warlike in bygone days, fighting the invading Fulanis from Sokoto in an attempt to retain their own land, only to be overcome later by those who had established the Emirate of Kontagora. Many of the Kamberri men nowadays joined the army and the pastor's wife was doing her best to teach the women household skills covered by the term Home Economics in the language of the USA, domestic science in English. Neither term is really suitable in the context of this teaching; possibly 'household management' is a better term. The pastor himself was trying to improve the local sanitation of the compounds around the mission but admitted he was more interested in horticulture and fruit production. He was trying without success to interest the Kamberri in eating the fruit he was trying to sell to them. Notably, he was not trying to teach them to grow fruit trees in their own compounds, although the soil and climate were ideal for this purpose.

(Anticipating somewhat, four months later, in the rainy season and at 2 a.m. I received a message in Bida which had come by 'cleft stick' from the mission near Auna, via Kontagora to Zunguru and by phone from Zunguru to Bida saying the missionary's child, now aged six months, was very ill with a high fever. I always thought of the possibility of cerebral malaria under such conditions, although I knew the infant had been given liquid quinine from birth. Therefore I packed my medical bag, left Bida at 3 a.m. and drove the 140 miles to Kontagora and told Dick Greswell (the DO) I was going to the Auna Mission, and why. The roads were bad as far as Ibeto but I managed to reach the village where I commandeered a bicycle which I rode ten miles, until the track became too bad, then a horse for the ten miles remaining. At 3.30 p.m., having pushed the rather refractory mare hard, I found the missionary hanging over his gate, chewing a straw. He said, 'Hello, how are you?' to which I replied, 'Let me see the child at once.' He chewed for a while, then said, 'I reckon the child was only teething. She is okay now.' This maddened me so I pushed past him and found the mother and child — temperature normal but undoubtedly teething. I took a blood smear, demanded a glass of his grapefruit juice which he had not offered me, and rode, cycled and motored back to Kontagora where Dick Greswell gave me a few stiff drinks to sooth my shattered composure then dinner and I found Chikizi with my bed in the ADO's house. I took the blood smear to the dispensary next morning and Mallam Isa Likita and I examined it under the microscope. It was negative for Plasmodium falciparum, much more serious than the benign tertian malaria (Plasmodium vivax) of India and the Far East.)

After another night in Auna we set off for Kontagora, where I was bidden to discuss medical and public health problems with Sarkin Sudan, the Emir. This took up most of the afternoon and early evening. He was a very shrewd but entertaining man, fond of a joke. Later in my first tour I got to know him much better. On my return to the rest house in the government station I was lucky to meet the Deputy Chief Conservator of Forests, Mr

D. R. Rosevear, an Oxford graduate. I told him I had noticed many differences in the vegetation between Bida (approximately 9° N and 6° E) and Zuru (11.5° N and 5° E). He was kind enough to give me a map of Nigeria showing the different ecological and vegetation zones, which he believed affected to a very great extent the nature of the diets eaten throughout the country. Apart from an unqualified study of the foods consumed by the Hausa and Fulani peoples living in and around Kano City (McCulloch, 1930) he was unaware of any systematic food consumption work on a quantative basis which had been carried out in Nigeria, and suggested that a food consumption survey based on the ecological zones would be of great value to the agricultural and forestry development programmes. Mr Rosevear also told me that 'considerable amounts of food were derived from the wild indigenous trees throughout the different ecological regions. His views interested me considerably. I kept an eye open for the different trees he mentioned. Also, instead of only visiting the dispensaries in the small towns, I visited the markets to see what locally grown foodstuffs were on sale. I found that nearly all the foods available to purchasers were indigenous, apart from imported salt, and in the larger markets, lump sugar.

We returned from Kontagora to Bida by a different route in order to cover the south-western part of my medical area. This included a dressing station and market at Bokani, and dispensary and markets at Mokwa and Kutigi. Preparations were being made at Mokwa for the mechanical ploughing of land for the production of groundnuts and food crops. It was fashionable in 1947/48 for the Colonial Development Corporation (CDC) to try to introduce mechanical means to spare the native populations the labour of hand-hoeing the land at the time of the year they were beginning to run short of food from last year's harvest in order to increase the yield of cash crops, mainly groundnuts and cow-peas, but in some areas cotton and rice. Attlee's UK government and the CDC did not have any conception of the difficulties, meteorological, geographical, ecological, agronomic or ethnic in the tribal sense, socio-economic and psychological, involved in changing the habits of people living for thousands of years more or less satisfactorily at subsistence level, the populations being kept in balance with their environments by the four horsemen of the Apocalypse — famine, flood, pestilence, and war. In *Before the Winds of Change* Bill Berry lists some of the CDC projects which were complete failures — the infamous groundnut scheme in Tanganyika, which cost the British taxpayer £335 million; the Nyasaland rice scheme; the Gambia egg scheme, costing £825,000, closed down in 1951 as did the Gambian rice/groundnut project, started by Berry himself under the direction of Professor B. S. Platt in 1947. Platt at that time was head of the Medical Research Council's worldwide nutritional activities and worked with the Gambian government through the Colonial Office, Creech-Jones being the Secretary of State for the Colonies. The Mokwa Mechanical Ploughing Scheme, started at the end of 1947, went the same way into oblivion. With hindsight I am sure the reason for these costly failures was lack of information on the disciplines listed above, but more importantly because they were pushed forward full speed at full scale without consultation with, and the co-operaiton of, the local people in the conduct of much smaller preliminary feasibility studies.

On our return journey to Bida, Joan Foster and I covered nearly 300 miles in the Bida NA lorry. Between the dispensary at Kutigi and Bida was the ferry at Wuya over the Kaduna River. This consisted of a planked deck large enough to take a three-ton lorry or two average-sized cars, floated on a number of forty-four-gallon petrol drums, its motive force coming from six to ten strong Nupe paddlers or polers. In the dry season when the river was low, about 100 yards across and the current comparatively sluggish it was easy for six men to pole the ferry almost directly across the river which had low, flattish banks on the west side with a concrete landing stage, but high, twenty foot, banks on the east or Bida side, down which an incline had been cut to a landing stage. In the wet season the river rose and flooded the west bank so that the total width would be sometimes over 200 yards and landing was carried out from the deck of the ferry via sturdy planks reaching out to the nearest piece of high ground firm enough to carry the weight of the vehicles. The expert ferrymen would pull the raft upstream by ropes to a point from which they reckoned that by strenuous paddling all ten of them could cross the river diagonally and fetch up at the landing stage. On many occasions when the water was high this worked satisfactorily for me. Only once in my experience did they miscalculate and my wife and son, my car and I were swept downstream until we touched the bank at a bend in the river three miles below the Bida-side landing stage. The technique then was for seven of the ten men to disembark and take a line with them on to the bank and pull the craft and contents upstream, the three men left on board poling the ferry away from snags on the bank. On that occasion missing the landing stage and the subsequent haul upstream added four hours to the time our journey would normally have taken.

In several trees on the Bida side of the ferry were large colonies of weaver birds (*Ploceidae*). They made a great noise building their bag-shaped covered nests and tending their young.

In the river, hippo and crocodiles could be a nuisance at low water, but not during the rains. While crocodile bites were often admitted to Bida hospital and to certain of the dispensaries, my family and I never had any trouble during the course of many crossings. In the Hausa language 'kada' means one crocodile; 'kadu' means a pair, and 'Kaduna' is the collective noun for crocodiles. The river of crocodiles, the Kaduna, runs through the town of Kaduna, hence the general hospital there was seldom without several examples of the damage which they can do to unwary people washing clothes on its banks, or fishing and swimming.

During the course of this first tour of 610 miles I had visited eight of my fifteen dispensaries and three of the nineteen dressing stations in the Bida medical area. They all seemed to me to be well staffed with dispensary attendants, midwives and dressers recruited from local people trained in Bida hospital or Kaduna. I had been fortunate to meet Dr Rosevear who had whetted my appetite and interest in respect of ecological and vegetation zones and the relationship between agricultural production, forestry, food consumption and health.

Food Consumption and Clinical Studies

I was now keen to start on the Etsu's suggestion to examine the prisoners' diet and extend this study to include the diets of the boys boarding in the middle school and to the 'pauper patients' diet in the Bida hospital. As I have said above Mallam Abubakar Zukogi Bida and I developed a methodology for measuring food consumption. We started by observation of the *status quo* before attempting anything quantitative.

The Colonial Office had warned me to take out to Nigeria my textbooks on the major subjects of medicine, surgery, obstetrics and tropical medicine and anything else I thought might be useful. Thus in addition to the major textbooks on clinical subjects which I had used as an undergraduate I had Grey's *Anatomy*; Dunlop, Davidson and McNee's *Textbook of Medical Treatment*; Davidson and Anderson's *Textbook of Dietetics*; Schadfer's *Physiology in Health and Disease*; Cole's *Dietetics in General Practice*; and Platt's *Tables of Representative Values of Foods commonly used in Tropical Countries* and a copy of the first (1943) edition of the American Medical Association's *Handbook of Nutrition.*

When we had found how foods were cooked and distributed among the prisoners and that guinea corn flour (Sorghum sativa) and rice (Oryza glaberrima) were the staple foods, supplemented by cowpeas (Vigna unguculata) and a soup containing small amounts of goat meat or beef, red palm oil (from Elaeis guineensis), pounded dried baobab leaves (Adamsonis digitata), fresh red peppers (Capsicum frutescens), okra (hibiscus sabdariffa) and salt (imported sodium chloride, not ionised), we weighed the edible portion of the different ingredients of the diet before and after they were cooked and the portions distributed to each consumer, namely twenty prisoners selected because they were clinically and biochemically found to be apparently healthy. The study lasted seven days. From the information obtained it was possible to calculate the energy and nutrient content of the diet using Platt's Tables. By comparison with a diet believed to be adequate (Platt, 1946) and with the clinical features shown by the subjects, it was hoped that any marked energy or nutrient deficiencies would be disclosed and a guide obtained to supplement or adjust the diet towards a better state of nutrition. The cost of the prison diet per head per day was calculated from current prices in the Bida market to be 2.85 pence (d) per head per day. Comparison with Platt's dietary objectives (1946) showed that energy and protein intake were ample for moderate activity, which was judged to be a fair description of the prisoners' work. It provided only half the recommended amount of riboflavin, two-thirds of that for ascorbic acid and half the amount of calcium. Signs of riboflavin deficiency were evident, angular stomatitis and sore tongues, but no obvious clinical features of scurvy or calcium deficiency were noted. These nutrient deficiencies could be overcome by the addition of two eggs (local hen's or guinea fowl's) and 250 ml of milk per day at an extra cost of 1.5d per day per head, a sum not acceptable to the NA Treasury. However, it was not the quantity and quality of the diet about which the prisoners were complaining, but the monotony of the same food every day. Hence it was eventually decided to everyone's satisfaction to vary the staple foods by this partial substitution from time to time, on an iso-calorie basis, of guinea corn and rice by yams (Dioscorea spp) or sweet potatoes (Ipomoea batatas) and the meat by twice the amount by weight of local dried fish which cost less than the meat ration and supplied more animal protein of good quality. Further variety was achieved by including a wider selection offresh vegetables in the soup, such as wild spinach (Amaranthus caudatus — *alayafu*) which cost nothing, because the prisoners were told to collect it from the surrounding bush; garden egg (Solaneum incanum — *gauta*), pumpkin (Cucurbita pepo — *kabewa*), locust bean cake (Parkin filicoidea — *daudawa*) and others.

The Bida Hospital 'pauper' diet was supplied by the Bida NA, not by the Medical Department so cost was important. It was more varied than the prison diet, the staple foods again being guinea corn and rice, but the soup contained either meat or fish, supplementary items being groundnuts (Arachis hypogaea) and bambara nuts (voandzeia subterranea); the soup, in addition to meat and fish, included onions and a wide variety of fresh leaves, powdered baobab leaf and red palm oil, the last two ingredients providing very large amounts of beta-carotine, precursor of vitamin A. The food consumption of twenty-five adults (male and female) was measured daily for one week, using the same methods described above to determine the prisoners' food intake. The diet was adequate in protein and calories and only riboflavin and calcium did not reach Platt's allowances. Again it was not difficult to eliminate those deficiencies without resort to the addition of milk and eggs, which were available in the markets but cost too much for the Treasury to support. Of the ordinary farmer or artisan living in Bida almost all had sore lips or tongues but clinical features of calcium deficiency were not observed.

The diets of twenty boys aged fourteen to sixteen years living in the Middle School dormitory were weighed and their food consumption was determined by the methods described above. (With some refinements regarding weighing the cooked and uncooked foodstuffs, these methods were continued throughout the many food consumption studies we undertook later throughout the whole of Nigeria. By now I had appointed an assistant to work with Mallam Abubakar, a nursing orderly; he also was a Nupe, Mallam Aliyu Bida, who had shown interest when we were measuring the hospital diet. Clinical examinations of all the fifty-seven boys dining in the boarding house were carried out. All of the twenty boys whose diets were studied appeared to be healthy apart from sore lips in ten of them. The diet provided was very similar in pattern to that of the hospital, being nutritionally adequate by Platt's standards in all respects except for riboflavin and calcium. The staple guinea corn and rice was bought at Bida Treasury controlled prices, the rest being bought at prices agreed between the Treasury and certain traders dealing with staple foods on a large scale. It cost 2.5d per head per day in February 1947. In common with the hospital diet it provided only 0.9 mg per head per day of riboflavin, Platt's objective being 1.8 mg and only 500 mg of calcium, the target being 800 mg per head per day.

As opposed to the 'captive' subjects in the prison and hospital we soon found that middle school boys were very liable to pick up bits and pieces of food in addition to the school diet when they paid visits to the town. We explained carefully to the twenty boys whose diets were being measured that they should report to M. Aliyu and M. Abubakar the sort and approximate amount of foods eaten outside school. M. Aliyu was asked to supervise and report on this habit, which were mainly sweetmeats and sugar, and did not significantly affect the overall dietary picture, except for a small increase in energy intake. However, we had learnt a lesson, which, in some subsequent surveys, made a considerable difference to the overall pattern and nutrient composition of diets, namely always to observe directly if possible, indirectly if necessary by questioning, what foods were eaten that day outside the home compound.

The Bida NA said they would be willing to invest up to an additional 1d a day per head in order to have as healthy and 'mentally alert' pupils as possible at the school. (One penny, the pound sterling then being at par with the West African pound and worth 240d.) This was largely due to the efforts of one of Etsu Nupe's senior councillors, Makaman Bida, an ex-headmaster of the Middle School. By juggling around with the foodstuffs locally available at what I considered reasonable cost, I came up with the following partial solution. By withdrawing 50 g of guinea corn and 75 g of rice from the established diet and adding one local hen's or guinea fowl's egg plus 125 ml of cow's milk, 15 g dried fish, 50 g of groundnuts, and 300 g of mangoes (as bought, not edible portion) or of guavas or paw-paw (as bought) the diet would provide 1,000 mg calcium and 1.4 mg of riboflavin at an extra overall cost of 1.1d. It was impossible to attain the full objective of 1.8 mg riboflavin without overshooting the Treasury's offer by more than it would provide. However, the Council agreed to the extra 0.1d over and above its original offer and put the new diet into effect forthwith. At the end of a year on the new diet the prevalence among those schoolboys of sore lips and tongues had fallen by 50 per cent. The headmaster would not hazard a guess about the increased alertness or learning ability!

Now we had to try our hands at gathering information from the local peasant farmers about their food production and consumption and to compare their energy and nutrient intake with their state of health. I was afraid that the peasant farmers' wives would resent the interference in their daily lives caused by our methods of measuring food consumption and that the women would object, or refuse, to be examined by me when they did not have any medical complaint. The population, about 100 persons in all, of the small hamlet we chose four miles outside the walls of Bida on the west side, called Kangi, was Nupe and pagan. The latter fact made it easier to do physical examinations on the women, but I always took with me one of the hospital midwives for their reassurance. Mallam Abubakar explained the reasons for our investigation to the headman of the hamlet in his own language (Nupe) and he did not raise any objections to our investigations of his farming methods or the women's cooking and marketing activities.

For the first period of seven days both Mallams lived in the village, one weighing the uncooked and cooked food and its distribution to all adults, the other following the men and women into the fields observing what they ate outside the home. The midwife accompanied the women if and when they went to the market in Bida. There the midwife observed what foodstuffs the women sold and what they bought, making as good an estimate of the amounts and prices paid for both boought and sold foodstuffs. She also noted what the women ate while at the market. She also weighed all the children under the age of two years living in the hamlet.

At this early stage in our investigations we recorded the food consumption of the farmers (over the age of twelve years) adding together and averaging the amounts eaten by men and women. The duration of each study was limited to seven days. After we had amassed more experience we found that it was easily possible to differentiate the amounts eaten by men, women and by children in the age groups four-six years and seven-twelve years as these age groups ate from different calabashes. Up to the age of four years we found that the sources of food, including breast feeding, were so various that it was not possible to be at all exact in recording the food intakes of the smaller children. We eventually discovered that the people included in a survey were liable to eat rather more in the first day or two of their study to 'show off' and again to eat more than usual during the last day of the food-weighing because they were glad to get rid of us. Thus it became the habit of the Federal Nutrition Unit (when it was formed in 1953) to weigh and measure food consumption for ten days at a time, discarding the first two and the last days' records using the middle seven days to obtain an average day's intake at any particular season of the year.

The first Kangi study at the beginning of March 1947 showed a quite different pattern of food consumption to that of the institutions studied in February. The staple foods were guinea corn and yams (Dioscorea), supplemented by items like cow-peas (Vigna) and cassava flour. The soup contained beef and fish, fresh and dried leaves, including dried baobab leaf, locust bean cake, fresh and dried red peppers (Capsicum) and salt. Considerable amounts of the edible portion of mangoes and some wild figs were the only fruits consumed. Apart from meat and fish, palm oil and salt, all the dietary ingredients were grown by the farmers themselves or gathered in the surrounding bush.

At current Bida market prices the cost of the complete diet would have been 1.9d. On a basis of per head consumed, the price of the items bought in the market averaged red palm oil 0.24d, beef 0.13d, fish 1.05d, imported salt 0.14d — total 0.56d. They were never paid for in cash but by bartering some of the produce brought to the market by the women of Kangi, for they were at a nearly absolute state of subsistence farming. When coin of the realm was needed to pay the 'head' tax determined from year to year by the NA Authorities working in co-operation with British government officials, the subsistence farmers would sell what farm produce they did not need themselves, e.g. a surplus of groundnuts, cowpeas and other agricultural produce specially grown for the purpose. If a more important matter, such as 'bride price', had to be found by a family this could be in the form of goats, sheep or, under certain circumstances, a small bit of land which carried a baobab tree or something equivalently productive as a means of barter. In the northernmost parts of the Bida medical area, cattle and agricultural 'cash crops' such as groundnuts and cotton were used for such special occasions.

In Bida town other sources of cash income were brass work and glass beads locally produced. In the late 1940s the Department of Statistics in Lagos believed that at least 80 per cent of the whole population of Nigeria lived at the level of subsistence farming such as that found at Kangi, and that this percentage might be higher in the Northern Province than in the Eastern and Western Regions.

The diet consumed by the adults farming around the hamlet of Kangi in March 1947, although more varied than those of the institutions, provided enough energy and protein to meet Platt's objective for moderately active people and using an allowance of 1 g protein from mixed sources per kg body weight per day. However, as in the case of the prison, school and hospital diets the two deficiencies found were of riboflavin and calcium. We had shown that these shortages could be put right, at least on paper, by adding milk and eggs to the schoolboys' diet. But as milk and eggs were 'cash crops' to the subsistence farmers, they could not afford to eat them, not because of any dislike of these foods but because the wealthier non-farming people in Bida, from the Etsu himself down to the 'expatriate' Ibo and Yoruba clerks and merchants in the government and NA service, as well as the few British expatriates living in the government station outside the town, were willing to pay what the local farmers considered a good price for them. Such a source of cash was normally spent by the subsistence farmer in Bida emirate on items like woven cotton cloth and other non-agricultural products he could not obtain from his own land. The same pattern was found to apply in Wushishi, Kontagora and Zuru, in fact throughout the Northern Province.

Of course the land was not always the farmer's own. His family may have lived on it for several generations but it belonged to the Etsu or one of the other of the three 'royal' families from which the Emir of Bida was always appointed by the 'Traditional Selectors'. Other people owned land and received produce from it. For instance, Makaman Bida, not of any royal Nupe house but educated at Katsina Secondary School and ex-headmaster of the Bida Middle School, presently a senior NA councillor, whose birth language was Nupe and whose Hausa and English were fluent and beautifully spoken, owned several farms on the south side of the town on the Jima road. He was broad-minded enough 'in the interests of agricultural development and nutritional knowledge' to allow his nephew, my Mallam Abubakar Zukogi Bida, to weigh and measure the adults' diets eaten in his own compound and we found it met and surpassed in all energy and nutrient aspects the 'objectives' set by Platt for the nutrition of colonial peoples (1946) and those of the American Medical Association Council on Foods and Nutrition (1946) for American citizens. The 'Makaman diet', as M. Abubakar and I called it between ourselves, was never reported to the SDC, Medical HQ, Lagos, or elsewhere, but it included plentiful amounts of eggs and milk, hence the lack of deficiencies of riboflavin and calcium.

In all the diets studied, guinea corn supplied ample quantities of thiamin, nicotinic acid and iron. The fresh leaves, fruit, sweet potatoes, red palm oil, and dried baobab leaves provided sufficient amounts of iron and ascorbic acid (vitamin C) and the precursor of vitamin A. The energy value of all diets was adequate to meet the requirements of moderately active adults. Although only 4 per cent of the total protein in the various diets studied in the Bida area was derived from animal sources, the intake was adequate at the level of 1 g of protein per kg per day from mixed vegetable and animal sources.

Food Consumption Studies — Application of Results obtained in Bida

As a result of the above observations I wrote a report to the DMS in Lagos, with copies to the Resident of Niger Province, at that time Mr Bryan Sharwood-Smith (later to become Governor of Northern Nigeria) and to the SDO of Bida Division, Mr Paul Brandt, who had replaced the unco-operative SDO who was stationed in Bida when I arrived. Paul Brandt was married but his wife seldom came to Nigeria because they had children at home in UK. He was keen on 'development' of all sorts, in particular agriculture and forestry.

In this report I included the following preliminary considerations — 'The Middle School boys should look after a small herd of cattle (bought by the NA and presented to the headmaster) which should provide eighteen gallons of milk per day, and if looked after by the boys themselves as part of their training, should cost very little. Eggs would be more difficult to supply in large quantities but a Middle School chicken farm might go far towards producing them. Groundnuts could be grown and stored by the boys and used as a cash crop to defer expenses. Fish could be produced by the construction of fish ponds on the Lanzu stream where it is swampy outside the east wall of the town, as it is done in the Doko area on the Kaduna river twelve miles south of Bida towards Pategi (a village on the Niger river). In fact . . . more intensive agricultural work could be carried out by the boys themselves, possibly to the detriment of their book learning but to the great benefit of their health (and possibly to their capacity to learn) and future usefulness as farmers.'

This preliminary report, well documented with tables of food intakes and costs at market prices, was well received in Lagos and by the Resident and District Officers who read it. The administrative officers advised that such studies should be extended to the Kontagora and Zuru areas where the staple food pattern would be different for ecological reasons and that food consumption should be measured at three monthly intervals to cover the different seasons of the year. In March, when the first Kangi survey had been done they considered the availability of food to be beyond its annual peak; that it would be at its lowest in May during the planting and growing seasons of the major food and cash crops, and highest between September and December, falling off gradually as the stores of harvested food were either eaten too quickly or over-sold to wealthy traders dealing in staple food products.

I next started to organise food consumption surveys in the Kontagora and Zuru areas, the first studies to be carried out if possible in March or early April 1947, and then in July/August, October and December 1947. I then handed them over to Mallams Abubakar and Aliyu for practical training in the prison and in Kangi, where they learnt how to measure food consumption and to observe and report what foods were eaten outside the compounds in addition to the diets prepared in the family kitchen. This was indeed a great advance.

CHAPTER 6

Family Interlude

From December 1946 when I sailed for Nigeria, Mary was having a rotten time in West Lodge, Fleet. She had taken a paying guest called Norah (neither of us can remember who or what she was, apart from being permanently in arrears in paying her rent). It was a cold snowy winter. When the snow melted the roof leaked and when the frost let up the frozen pipes were found to be cracked and they leaked. She was doing her best to get a passage to Nigeria for herself and C. but this became complicated when first C. and then she went down with mumps.

The opportunities for passage to Nigeria seemed to vary from ocean transport in the autumn to a new route recently developed by BOAC, flying York bomber aircraft converted for passenger travel which flew from Heathrow to my old staging post on the way home from India, Castel Benito in Libya by day, then across the Sahara in the cool of the night to Kano, Northern Nigeria. After many uncertainties and disappointments she made a firm booking for 16 March, arriving in Kano early next morning. She and C. were each allowed 60 lbs. weight of luggage, a generous allowance. She had never flown before and was a bit scared by the whole idea. But when faced with such situations she is always very courageous.

She and Christopher arrived in Kano then went on to Zunguru by train where I met them in the Bida NA three-ton lorry. By now its driver and I were quite good friends and I had picked up a word or two of Hausa. The sixty-mile drive to Bida took about two hours and we arrived at our bungalow in the Bida government station around 9 p.m. Mary and C. were exhausted but the sight of the beautifully red-cardinal polished floor of the sitting room and dining room, Chikizi in spotless white uniform with a tray of drinks including fresh grapefruit juice from our own small orchard made them feel better and ready for some soup and roasted guinea fowl cooked by Bernard, the cook-boy. We had two bedrooms in that bungalow, one with a single PWD bed for C. and a double-bed for us, with mosquito-nets which intrigued C., as had a genuine 'punkah' for over the dining-table which was moved by a rope passing through the wall. He did not see Azuzu that evening, who provided with his toe the motive power for the punkah. Azuzu was appointed C.'s 'boy' from the next day, and in fact looked after our daughter also in the years to come. When C. wanted to go for a walk, Azuzu was always in front of him, guarding against snakes or other small denizens of the ten-foot-high elephant grass which in many places bordered the paths along which they walked — often to see one of Azuzu's friends who worked in one or other of the few European compounds.

Mary settled in quickly and soon had the boys and cook working well for her. Bernard did the marketing and as he knew I was keeping in close touch with market prices, the list of cash expenditures he brought to Mary daily for checking with the goods he bought was always correct. Christopher was fascinated by our water boy because he had a very large and prominent umbilical hernia; Mary was amazed at the expertise of the washerman who cleaned the clothes so well using only 'bar-soap' and ironed them with a charcoal iron.

An important chore which I handed over to Mary was the drill for filtering and boiling all water before it was used for cooking or drinking. A filter cupboard was part of the PWD furniture in all houses occupied by government staff. This cupboard was used to contain one's own filter consisting of an upper container for about one gallon of water, which then passed through a Berkfelt filter candle into a lower chamber, whence we took it to the kitchen for boiling before decanting it into jugs for drinking purposes, or the cook used it in the preparation of meals. The filter candle had to be removed, washed and boiled once a week and replaced about every six months. Many people did it the other way round, i.e. boiled then filtered the water and this could lead to trouble if the candle and its retaining washers were in any way faulty or dirty.

The main bit of equipment we lacked in our own bungalow was a refrigerator. However, the large locally made earthenware jars did quite a good job at cooling such items as butter, which came weekly from the train at Zunguru sixty miles away in an ex-army pack carried on the back of a sweating cyclist, and bottles of beer. In the dry season the cooling jars worked better than during the rains, but then the temperatures were lower. So we all settled down well until the time came to do our first tour *en famille*.

Food Consumption Studies — extension to Kontagora and Zuru

Again we all packed into the Bida NA three-tonner, 'loads' (baggage, including personal and technical equipment, boys and the two Mallams Abubakar and Aliyu. We were to meet the personal of the Field Medical Unit at Kontagora, where they were not wasting their time but doing a morbidity survey in the town.

With the help of the Emir of Kontagora I selected a small hamlet of similar size to Kangi and the Emir explained to the people the objectives of the food consumption and clinical examinations in which they would be expected to co-operate. This was an excellent way to start our survey and the people did not cause us any trouble — in fact they became interested in knowing the results of our work. The village selected was called Tunga Wawa about six miles from the Kontagora market, the inhabitants were pagan Hausa-speaking people of Kanberri origin who had been conquered by the Fulani two centuries ago. All were settled farmers and a few owned one or two Zebu cattle.

The first part of the Kontagora food consumption and clinical survey was carried out in early April 1947, for seven days. As in the case of the first Kangi (Bida) investigation (March 1947) it was carried out when preparations such as hoeing and bush clearing were being done, before the rains and the sowing of the millet sorghum started. After the food consumption work was in hand at Tungan Wawa I left Mallam Aliyu and five members of the Field Medical Unit there and went on up to Zuru with Mallam Abubakar and the rest of the Field Medical Unit to make arrangements for a similar survey near that village. Mr 'Nicky' McClintock was the ADO Zuru at the time and he introduced me to the chief of the Zuru Federation. The people in this area are pagans of the Dakakerri tribe. Even in times of peace almost all the young males do a period of service with the WAAF, and the Dakakerri women lose face if they marry a man who has not been in the army. In April 1947 many of the younger farmers had not long been demobilised after serving part of the war in Burma and were glad to be back in their homes and with home-grown food and with their own women. As in UK a 'population bulge' was in the making at this time in the Zuru chiefdom.

I selected a hamlet two miles west of Zuru for our survey, again with the help of the Chief. He was not as enthusiastic about the scheme as the Emir of Kontagora but did not raise any objections and told his people to co-operate, which they did. So we established three food consumption and clinical surveys in Niger Province designed to take place:
(a) while the land was being cleared and/or hoed for sowing before rains were expected to start at the end of April or early May;
(b) in July/August when the bulrush millet (pennisetum-*geo*) should be ripe towards the end of the rains; and
(c) in November/December when the guinea-corn should be harvested.

The growth of other food and cash crops, which would also vary with the seasons, including cowpeas (Vigna), yams, leaves of baobab trees, okra, mangoes, groundnuts and cotton, were observed. That year (1947) the rains came at the usual time, there was no drought and everyone agreed that the production of food and cash crops was average to good.

Kangi and Tungan Wawa lie respectively in the southern and northern areas of the ecological zone known as *Guinea savannah* and that Zuru is in the heart of *Sudan savannah* zone. The differences in the types of food crops produced and eaten in the three areas is considerable, and these differences are reflected in the pattern of nutrient intakes, as will be discussed later.

All the occupants of the hamlets where food consumption studies were carried out were examined physically, weighed and clinical signs which might be attributed to lack of specific nutrients were recorded. The Filed Medical Unit staff examined blood, urine and faeces for evidence of infestations and I determined haemoglobin levels and presence or absence of urobilinogen in the urine as a possible indicator of impaired liver function.

The midwife at the Zuru dispensary was a very competent young woman who became interested in food consumption in relation to the health of her pregnant patients and their new-born children. I managed to get her a set of scales (yard-arm) and taught her how to use them and how to prepare a graph of monthly weight for age for each child. By the end of the year's food survey activities she had recorded 813 monthly weights from 176 infants born during that period who had been brought regularly to the dispensary.

Life in the Government Reservation, Bida
The full European population of Bida amounted, at any given time, to between eight and twelve people, depending upon who was away on tour or on leave, so this was too small a number to warrant a social club. Apart from going around from house to house for evening drinks before dinner we mainly met our fellow expatriates in the afternoons on the tennis courts, where everyone foregathered, most to play, some only to gossip.

A young fig tree beside the courts gave shade from the sun for spectators and for players between games. At certain times of the year, if one sat very quietly under this tree, it was possible to hear thousands of caterpillars munching the leaves. These caterpillars were popular as a soup ingredient among the villagers throughout Niger Province.

The Europeans living in Bida hired a number of Zebu cattle from Fulani herdsmen who had settled in the vicinity of the town using areas for grazing specified by the NA council. The milk provided by this small herd was brought in bulk to a volunteer at whose compound the 'small boys' from other houses gathered at 6 a.m. to receive their master's quota. Mary, as the MO's wife, was in duty bound to undertake this chore which involved straining the raw, and often still warm, milk through muslin to remove the flies, bits of grass and other undesirable additives, and then measure and distribute the amounts requested. She paid the Fulani one penny (1d) a pint and kept records of amounts issued to each consumer. Any surplus milk sold to the Middle School at the same price, which was a little less than that prevailing in the Bida market. Needless to say all the consumers of this milk knew that it must be boiled and then simmered for twenty minutes and stored in a refrigerator or cooling jar. Once a month the milk club accounts were settled beneath the fig tree beside the tennis courts.

Food Consumption, Health and Agriculture —
Further Developments
A Provincial Development Committee was asked to meet in

FAMILY INTERLUDE

Minna for four days in May 1947. The committee was charged with the task of co-ordinating the work of the administration, governmental and NA with that of the different technical services with particular emphasis on the remote areas rather than on Provincial HQ or one or two of the more favoured areas. New schools and dispensaries, fresh fruit tree nurseries, maintenance and improvement of market stalls and slaughter slabs, local irrigation schemes, new wells, bridges and so on were all items encouraged to be placed on the agenda.

My activities in Bida, Kontagora and Zuru were commended by the Resident and the three chiefs concerned. I explained my ideas for extension of our food consumption, health, agricultural and forestry activities and these were approved in general and particularly by the Emir of Kontagora, provided the expenses could be kept to a minimum agreed by the NA. The committee proposed close co-operation between me and the agricultural, veterinary and forestry officers in future developments and called upon the Chief Commissioner of the Northern Region (Sir John Patterson) to rekindle the activities of the Regional Nutritional Committee. All this was very satisfactory. On return to Bida I continued working at the hospital, touring the southern areas of my district and drawing up a plan for Kontagora to start as soon as possible.

Food Production and Consumption —
Kontagora Trial Village — Tungun Maidubu
I had sent a letter to my mother in Aberdeen saying that it would be nice if she could come and see how we lived in Africa. To our amazement two weeks later I received a telegram saying she would arrive at Kano airport on 23 August 1947. As I was already committed to the August/September food consumption survey in Kontagora and Zuru we would have to take mother with us. We met her at Zunguru station on 25 August, fitted her and her loads into our vehicles and set off for Kontagora where she stayed in the spare wing of Dick Greswell's house, and Mary, C. and I were again in the ADO's house.

I asked that Duncan McKinlay, the agricultural officer in Niger Province, join me in Kontagora on this trip for preliminary discussions with the Emir. The current fashion was that a piece of land would be cleared of scrub and trees, then hand-hoed before planting, weeded during the growing season and the crop harvested when ripe. This process was repeated year after year until the land became infertile, when it was allowed to lie fallow for some years and another area was cleared. Duncan McKinlay and I had worked out on paper that an average family in this area of Guinea savannah, a farmer with one or two wives and four to six children, could exist without moving from their village or hamlet, or walking to far-off fields, if each was based permanently upon fifteen acres of land, of which plenty was available. The Geological Survey Department considered that sufficient water could be obtained on a year-round basis from a well to supply six families between sixty and eighty feet deep, provided that severe drought was not encountered for more than three consecutive seasons. That department had plans to sink many wells to provide artesian water in the Northern Region, but so far money for this purpose had not been included in its annual budget. The Public Works Department stated they could construct one deep sub-soil water well capped, sealed and fitted with a pump adjustable to levels of water down to eighty feet for the use of several families. This was too good an offer to turn down and Dick Greswell explained to the Emir that this work would be carried out at no expense to the NA if he would arrange for the land needed to provide each of six families with fifteen acres near the existing village of Tungan Wawa, where the food consumption and clinical survey was taking place. Plenty of land was available.

Our idea was to divide the fifteen acres into strips radiating from the centre of the village, one strip being of five acres resting fallow on which three zebu cows would be grazed, the next five acres for growing the staple grain crops and vegetables such as beans, and the last five acre strip being reserved for cash crops, mainly groundnuts, cowpeas and cotton. Fruit trees would be grown around the compounds, mango, guava, (psidium Guava), pawpaw (carica papaya), and others; neem trees to produce shade on a short-term basis and fig trees for longer-term shade and fruit. The whole system would be subject to rotation, the cereal crops going to the area planted by cash crops and vice versa. Every two or three years the grazing area would be cleared and taken into the rotation pattern. The zebu cows, inoculated against rinderpest and other diseases, would be used for pulling ploughs of local construction made with the assistance of the provincial PWD for the metal share. Mr Daldy, Inspector of Works, Minna, had agreed to do this, gratis, during the Development Committee meeting. Both Duncan and I had realised that the mechanical farming being attempted at Mokwa to produce staple food and cash crops was foundering upon the inability of the local farmers, even with the help of the NA, to maintain the machinery involved and pay for the fuel to run it. Therefore we were convinced that any form of mechanical aids, such as tractors, should not be used to assist the farmers in their hardest task of the year, namely hoeing the ground. It would be preferable to use home-owned oxen to draw a plough, with the added advantage of the manure they would return to the soil. The ground was reasonably flat but a little contouring could be taught to prevent erosion.

We discussed the idea that September of 1947 with the Emir. He was much in its favour, particularly as it would cost the Kontagora NA very little — only six new compounds to be built by the local people themselves, a deep well with covers and pumps to be carried out by the Provincial Office of Works, and the provision of cattle, preferably cows that could be kept in milk. The new huts would be sprayed with DDT against flies (dysentery and typhoid) and mosquitoes (malaria). Great care would be taken to keep the surroundings of the well clear of puddles of water and the soil there as dry as possible to counteract the possibility of acquiring or passing on infestations by hook-worm (ankylostomiasis), bilharzia (anhistosomiasis) and guinea-worm (dracontiasis). The new hamlet would be called Tungan Maidubu, in honour of Umaru Maidubu, the Emir. He would ask for six families to volunteer to participate in the new venture. Later I was told by his eldest son that, from plentiful applications, his father had chosen a group of six families interested in mixed farming, as were we all. The proposal was approved by the Resident and the NA.

At the beginning of September 1947 we left Kontagora for Bida, having completed the food consumption and clinical work. On the return journey we visited the dispensaries at Rijau, Tegina and Zunguru. Meanwhile the Emir, Provincial Works Department and others involved, such as sanitary inspectors, got on with the initial preparatory work.

I added one important rider to the scheme. It should not be expanded in any way for at least six years from the inception of organised mixed farming and crop production on a rotation basis so that comparisons could be made between the 1947 levels of food consumption and clinical conditions and those prevailing in 1953 to determine whether or not the proposed Tungan Maidubu was a success or failure. It should be supported by NA funds during these six years.

My Mother's visit to Kano, Kontagora and Bida
It was something of a rarity in those days for European officers posted to 'bush' stations to have their wives in Nigeria with them; it was even rarer for a wife to bring out a five-year-old child with her, but it was unheard of for a grandmother to visit her grandchild, son and daughter-in-law. Mother proposed to stay with us for a month. As I have said we met her at Zunguru and had to take her with us on tour to Kontagora where she stayed in Dick Greswell's house. He was very kind to her, giving her a short history of the Fulani, Hausa and pagan tribes in Northern Nigeria. He arranged an audience for her with Sarkin Sudan who had never before met the mother of one of the Europeans working in his emirate. I recollect they laughed a great deal during their conversation, as parents will when discussing their children, provided they have 'turned out all right'. The Emir's eldest son was a serious young man who had been to Kalsina secondary school and spoke English and the old man was proud of him.

When we returned to Bida mother insisted on a visit to Etsu Nupe's palace and he allowed her to visit his *harem* but only accompanied by Mary, who by now was getting to know the drill whereby she would only visit the official wives and some of the senior concubines.

My mother had elected to go home via Lagos, where Carl Wilson would put her up for a few days before she flew back to London via Kano. We drove her to the extreme south-west corner of my medical area beyond Mokwa and into Jebba Town in Ilorin Province, across the railway bridge over the Niger past the island carrying the tall rock famous for its deadly swarms of African bees. We saw her into the train and later heard from her that she had a good journey to Lagos and flight to UK.

FAMILY INTERLUDE

The Development of Tungan Maidubu

The NA and PWD had started work energetically in September 1947. The land on which Tungan Maidubu was to be built had been lying fallow for many years and had already been cleared of trees and roots. It was now being cleared by hoe and the huts built. The well was sunk, covered and aproned, with a hand pump fitted. Some sorghum and millet had been planted, probably too late, zebu cattle had been provided for the six families chosen by the Emir, and things were going well. The ploughs were not yet ready for use but would soon be available when practice ploughing could be started.

While the food consumption and nutrition surveys were going on at Kangi (Bida), Tungan Wawa (Kontagora) and Zuru I did a lot of touring, mainly in the northern part of the medical area. Mary and C. often came with me on tour from Bida as far as we could take the car. Obviously if I had to visit some out of the way dispensary or dressing station by horse or bicycle for a night or two they stayed in Bida or in Kontagora.

In early November I was offered the chance to leave Bida and be based in Kontagora to continue on a full-time basis with the Tungan Maidubu development work and the completion of the surveys at Kangi, Tungan Wawa and Zuru.

By the beginning of December, when we moved to Kontagora, Mary was six months pregnant. All arrangements had been made for her to have the baby in Kano under the medical care of Dr Hall. She had played tennis in Bida until July and was very fit, so I was not at all worried about looking after myself until the calculated time for her to go into hospital.

Tungan Maidubu was fully occupied by early March 1948 and the first ploughing had been carried out by the end of March, ready for sowing the food crops and planting cash crops as soon as the rains started.

At the end of March, when Mary was due to go to Kano for her confinement, a telegram arrived from Joey Walker, DMS, ordering me to report immediately to Lagos to work there as physician in the General Hospital. His telegram had been sent by 'sounder' up the railway line to Zunguru and onwards to Kontagora over the last eighty miles by 'cleft stick'. I sent a lengthy reply saying that my wife was due to go to Kano any day now to have the baby under Dr Hall's care and could my posting to Lagos be postponed until my next tour. It was also important to supervise the Tungan Maidubu trial at least until June 1948 when I was due for leave. In reply I received a direct order to report to Lagos immediately and that an ambulance would meet us at Ebuta Metta station to take Mary to the Creek Hospital in Lagos where a bed was reserved and Dr Ian McGregor, the surgical and obstetrics specialist, would look after her. He also said that good hospitals and doctors were available at Ilorin, Ibadan and Abeckuta along the railway line, in case 'your wife is taken short *en route*'!

Sarkin Sudan, the Emir of Kontagora, was kind enough to lend us his large Chevrolet saloon car to drive Mary as softly as possible to Zunguru.

When we reached Ebuta Metta and ambulance was waiting for us. The driver told us that our future house in Ikoyi, 20 Glover Road, was still occupied by my predecessor and he was to take us to the Government Rest House in Ikoyi, near the hospital. Dr McGregor visited Mary the next day, found that all as well and reserved a bed for her at the Creek Hospital where European staff were treated.

After ten days in the Rest House we were able to move in to 20 Glover Road, and were rejoined by our own houseboys who were delighted to be back again in Lagos. The house was struck by lightning one night but even this event did not start any labour pains. At last Dr McGregor agreed to admit Mary to hospital and induce labour when she was three weeks overdue according to her calculations.

Mary produced our daughter Diana at 2.10 a.m. on 21 April 1948 before I had returned home from a dinner party. At 2.30 a.m. Dr McGregor came round to our house to tell me the good news of Diana's arrival and stayed an hour having a drink and gossiping about Edinburgh, telling me not to go to the hospital until 4 a.m. Eventually, after the Irish nursing sister in charge of Mary had given me some black coffee, I was allowed to see Mary and a small infant with a lot of jet black hair. Mary was annoyed because Diana only weighed 5 lbs. 10 ozs. in spite of the size she (Mary) had been and the three late weeks. She had insisted that this weight be checked but it was correct.

While we were living in the Ikoyi Government Rest House and while Mary was in the Creek Hospital I had made friends with a new recruit to the Nigerian Civil Service, Ronald Berriff, who had been in the Honourable Artillery Company pre-war. With the East Yorks he spent 1939-40 in France; Dunkirk; was then posted to the Bombay Grenadiers and served in India until transferred to the 7th Gurkhas and moved to Italy for the rest of World War II. Dick Greswell had been posted from Kontagora to the Secretariat in Lagos and he and Ron Berriff, both bachelors at that time, became great friends. Dick and Ron were frequent visitors to Glover Road to give Diana her evening bottle of Cow and Gate milk formula — as they said they needed the practice for the future. Dick was already engaged and was about to be married on his next leave. Ron was still at the stage of summing up the relative merits of the secretaries who worked in the secretariat building on the Marina.

Not long before we were due to go on leave I heard from the DO who had taken over from Dick Greswell in Kontagora that Max Backhouse, who had replaced Bryan Sharwood-Smith as Resident, Niger Province, was so impressed by the planning and operation of Tungan Maidubu trial, that he had decided to start four other similar settlements in spite of my caveat against such early expansion. The cost to the Kontagora NA for the additional plough shares, working cattle and digging of wells, would have added about four shillings per annum to the government-levied capitation tax of about £10 paid by each householder, a sum that the Emir was not willing to demand through the NA. This upset the activities we had planned and it would probably be impossible to assess the success or failure of the new hamlet. It was an example of the warning given to me by Dr Macnamara, my predecessor in Bida, of conflicting interests between government administration and native authorities which could often be disastrous in the area of agricultural development policy in relation to food production and nutrition. Such lack of co-operation is a common cause of failure of development programmes at higher national and international level.

So at the end of July 1948 Mary, C., Diana and I boarded the Elder Dempster mail boat *Accra* and reached Liverpool two weeks later, after a brief stop at Las Palmas in the Canary Islands.

CHAPTER 7

The Delta Province

First Leave from Nigeria
We were making for Edinburgh and a flat in the Morningside area of the city.

I spent much of our leave preparing a paper based on the food consumption and clinical data collected in Niger Province, at Bida, Kontagora and Zuru. This paper confirmed Don Rosevear's views that the staple and other food crops grown in different ecological and vegetation zones would have different nutritional values. It was published in the *British Journal of Nutrition* in 1949.

The energy value and mineral and vitamin composition of the diets consumed in Bida, Kontagora and Zuru were compared with Platt's 'Objectives for the Nutrition of Colonial Peoples' (Platt, 1946) and with the US National Research Council's recommended allowances for American citizens (Nutr. Rev. 1948).

The data acquired showed that the diets provided enough energy for both men and women to live a 'moderately' active life; the protein content of the diets was adequate, judged by a requirement of 1 g/kg body weight from mixed dietary sources, although the amount of animal protein consumed was very small.

Thus, in spite of a reasonably good diet, apart from the specific deficiencies mentioned above, only 45 per cent of all the people examined were categorised 'good', 46 per cent 'fair' and 9 per cent 'poor' as regards their general appearance. This finding was not surprising as 20 per cent had clinically demonstrable liver disease or had had attacks of jaundice, 6 per cent gave a history of haematuria and urobilinogen was present in the urine of 42 per cent of the subjects.

The above facts indicate the importance which must be given to public health and environmental sanitation measures in addition to improved agricultural productions and better food consumption if under-nutrition and malnutrition are to be eradicated.

Posting to Warri
We returned to Nigeria and to my new posting as MO at Warri, in February 1949. At that time Warri was the highest point on its creek in the Niger Delta, which could be reached by the sea-going vessels, where they had to moor out in the stream, cargo being loaded and unloaded onto lighters for transport to and from jetties.

The Warri posting was generally supposed to be a step up in the professional, as opposed to administrative, ladder of promotion in the Medical Department. I was surprised therefore when my predecessor seemed reluctant to leave but this soon became clear.

In Southern Nigeria, both east and west, the prevalence of yaws (framboesia), a contagious disease causing very unsightly skin rash on any part of the body caused by a spirochaete (treponema), akin to that causing syphilis, is very high. Skin lesions are found in many children but the infection may be acquired at any age. In the 1940s the intramuscular injection of organic arsenical drugs caused a very rapid improvement in the clinical features of the disease. Even one injection would lead to visible improvement and if given regularly at weekly intervals for some months, the condition could be cured. However, reinfection was always a possibility. It had been established custom until I reached Warri in 1949 that the MO journeyed around the medical area, stopping at certain predetermined places, e.g. under a particular fig tree or at an outlying dispensary, to inject the children and adults who came from the surrounding bush, with arsenical drugs. There were three such circuits in common use covering the more populous areas of the province. An elderly hospital orderly always accompanied the MO on those tours and, by bush telegraph, let it be known which of the three routes would be followed on any given day. As the injections were always given into the buttocks of children and adults, the practice had acquired the title of 'bum-punching'. Because patients under such irregular conditions could not properly be followed up with regular weekly injections, and because even one injection could cause considerable improvement, the practice of bum-punching was looked upon with disfavour by Medical Headquarters. Further, private practice by Colonial Service MOs when treating natives of the territory in which they worked was not allowed by the Colonial Office. Unfortunately, such was the demand for 'bum-punching' among the natives of Southern Nigeria that most medical officers took advantage of it, buying the arsenical drugs from medical stores and charging those suffering from yaws an exorbitant price per injection, a habit frowned upon by the Nigerian administration. The hospital orderly in Warri, Tete by name, had been given 10 per cent of the takings by previous MOs.

Now I can revert to the MO I was replacing. It was obvious that he was spending most of his time bum-punching and not attending the out-patient clinics whence should have come the African in-patients. He had not gained the confidence of the local Europeans or senior African civil servants, nor that of the European traders, who would normally use the hospital annex. He left three weeks after my arrival and I never heard of this obstructive character again in Nigeria or elsewhere.

Delta Province

This part of Nigeria was completely different from the Bida medical area. Delta Province covered an area of approximately 9,600 square miles and had a population in the late 1940s of about 800,000 people, a density of 83 persons per square mile, more or less uniformly distributed throughout the area of rain forest, fresh water swamp and mangrove swamp of which it was composed. The climate is hot and very humid throughout the year, the rainfall varying from 120 to 180 inches per annum, with little seasonal variation, compared to a mean of about 60 inches in Bida during the wet season (April/May to September/October), to half an inch in the dry season and 40 inches in Kontagora and Zuru in the rains and 0 inches in the dry weather. Thus in Delta Province little seasonal variation was found in planting of crops and in food consumption. Delta was the most easterly coastal province of the Western Region. The tribes occupying the northern part of the province were Isoko and Urhobo. In the mangrove swamps on the west side of the delta the predominant tribe was the Itsekeri (pronounced Jekeri) and on the east side were the Ijaw people. The Isoko and Urhobo farmed the fresh water swamp and the dry land in the rain forest zone; the Itsekeri and Ijaws were fishermen living on a series of islands in the salt water mangrove swamps.

THE DELTA PROVINCE

*Warri: Provincial Headquarters,
Delta Province*
Warri, when we were there in 1949, was a very happy station comprising a cross-section of all the expatriate types found in West Africa.

Warri was so isolated and the expatriate population of around thirty to forty people was so closely knit that misfits could not easily be tolerated and many who came had to be posted elsewhere by the administration or their employers. For those of us who made the grade Warri was a wonderfully interesting and worthwhile place in which to serve.

Warri Medical Area
The MO Warri was responsible for the whole of Delta Province. The Warri General Hospital had been very well built before the First World War. The MO's house was in the hospital compound. There were 200 beds in five wards, fifty of each for male medical and surgical patients, seventy-five for female medical and surgical cases and a maternity ward for twenty-five patients. Very often the last category were 'patients' rather than 'maternity cases' due to the widespread local custom of female circumcision which often inhibited normal dilation of the vulva during childbirth, necessitating surgery more complex than simple episiotomy, a minor precautionary intervention often required worldwide in women with normal genitalia if the baby's head is very large.

The Maples Annex had been built early in the century near the bank of the creek and was a very solid building raised on stilts about fifteen feet above ground level. It comprised ten single well-furnished rooms with individual washing and lavatory accommodation and a four-bedded ward for men. This senior service 'annex' had to deal with all the categories of patient mentioned above from both Delta and Benin Provinces. Just before I left Warri after a 24-month tour, X-ray equipment was installed on the ground floor of the annex and a radiographer added to the hospital establishment. The equipment appeared to be of good British quality but I was never able to use it as the radiographer had not appeared at the time of my departure.

Thus the NA dispensaries for which I was responsible appeared to be under more control from the administrative officers than from the NAs headed by their tribal chiefs. Dispensaries were located at Ughelli Divisional HQ, Awale District, Forcados District, and at Koko on the Benin River west of Sapele District. Apart from Forcados all these dispensaries could be reached by roads, mostly of very poor quality. For instance, the road to Awale from Ughelli was only a grassy track but I never found it impassable as it was well maintained and drained.

These dispensaries were staffed by attendants and midwives, trained at Warri Hospital. They relied on that hospital for medical supplies. Dressing stations as found in the north were not needed owing to the compactness of the province. Patients could be brought to dispensaries or hospitals by vehicle or by canoe if they could not walk or ride a bicycle. The high population density (83 per square mile) resulted in a much larger number of daily attendances at these four dispensaries and the hospital out-patient departments than in the much more extensive Bida medical area (population 23 per square mile).

Clinical Practice in Warri District (Medical)

Out-patient attendances were high soon after I had developed a routine which started daily, except Sundays, at 7 a.m. It was impossible to learn the many local languages spoken in the province and, although Yoruba was the official *lingua franca* of the region, few of the Itsekeri, Ijaw and Urhobo tribes spoke anything but their own languages, which were specific for each tribe and not dialects of Yoruba. Most of the African traders from these tribes living and working in Warri township spoke English. Thus I had to depend very largely upon interpreters in the out-patient clinics as I had had to do in the orderly room of Wellington Hospital in the Nigiri Hills, South India. The medical orderly Tete could speak a number of the major local languages as well as Yoruba, a language I am ashamed to say I never tried to learn.

Gradually the wards started to fill with patients who needed good nursing or, more often, surgery. The illnesses prevalent in the Delta Province were, on the whole, very similar to those encountered in the Bida medical area, tropical diseases as well as the types of illnesses found in temperate climates. There was some difference in the incidence of the tropical infections and infestations between Warri and Bida. Malignant tertian malaria was holoendemic in both areas. Unfortunately in Delta Province the malaria parasite was carried by a mosquito (Anopheles Gambiae) which had adapted to living in stagnant brackish or salt water in the mangrove swamps. Amoebic and bacillary dysentery were always with us, requiring careful administration of the necessary medicines which, if given in the wrong dosage, could be dangerous. Good nursing was the key to recovery of many patients suffering from dysentery, helped if need be by surgery for amoebic liver abscesses and intravenous saline drips to counter dehydration. Bilharzia (Schistomiasis haematobium and Mansoni) was very seldom encountered, and, as the local dwarf Muturu cattle were immune to trypanosomiasis, sleeping sickness was not a problem. On the other hand hook-worm (ankylostomiasis) and round-worm (ascariasis) infestations were more prevalent in the Warri area than in Bida. The filaria parasites (wuchereria bancrofti) which caused elephantiasis in Niger Province and had given me so much surgical practice there, were not found in Delta Province but in the latter area the two other filarial worms (*filaria loa-loa* and *onchocerca volvulus*) were common. Loa-loa infestation, from which I suffered myself for a few years until it died out, was only a nuisance when the adult worms migrated from place to place in the subcutaneous tissues causing the sensation known as formication, as if ants were crawling on one's skin, and occasionally a mild nettle-rash. Onchocerca volvulus, on the other hand, was a serious condition which could cause 'river blindness' if the larvae (microfilaria) of the adult worms damaged the conjunctiva, cornea, iris or the retina. Swelling of lymph nodes and an itchy rash were common symptoms. These larvae were carried from infected persons to others by a small fly, *simulium damnesum*, which lived in the grasses growing alongside running streams. In those days every effort was made by the sanitary inspectors and their staff to keep the banks clear of weeds and grass from above to below water level and to kill the flies' eggs by introducing solutions of copper sulphate into the streams at their sources, if possible. This approach to controlling the simulium fly was not effective. Suramin and diethylcarbamazine were not available in 1949 and treatment had to be palliative.

Leprosy was much more common in Warri than in the Bida medical area. Yaws was endemic, as I have described above, and

I found that the opinion of the staff of the hospital, and certainly that of Tete who stood to make some money from it, was on the whole in favour of the 'bum-punching' practice, as the out-patient department was less liable to become a focus for infection if the sufferers from the disease were treated elsewhere. It was a vexed question, particularly as the outlying dispensaries were not issued with the arsenical drugs used for the treatment of yaws and the dispensary attendants were not allowed to give injections. This I thought a short-sighted approach and so reported to the DMS. His reply was to the effect that, if the dispensary attendants gave injections of arsenic for yaws or penicillin for gonorrhoea (for which they would charge a fee), under-dosage of such medicines would occur resulting in bacterial resistance to the drugs. This made good sense and I compromised by doing only one day a week touring a circuit of about six assembly points for the purpose of 'bum-punching'. The circuit was the same every week so that regular injections would be possible and was chosen to cover areas of higher population density. This boring chore took place on Saturdays after I had finished with the out-patient department. The odd, or possibly not so odd, aspect of these weekly tours was that the patients insisted on paying for the injections, 'to make sure the medicine was proper and strong'. Tete got his 10 per cent of the takings!

Syphilis was not often seen in Delta Province and, if diagnosed, was treated with penicillin. Gonorrhoea was also teated by penicillin.

Another source of severely ill patients was injury from crocodile bites and, a new type of case for me, goring by the fierce and wily West African buffalo known as 'bush-cow'. The latter type of injury could be very serious as any of those bites or gorings was always liable to lead to tetanus or gas-gangrene, for which we gave anti-tetanus serum, hoping for no anaphylactic reactions, and penicillin by intramuscular injection.

The out-patient department stabilised at a very large number of attendances per day, more than could be handled satisfactorily by me and the nursing staff at morning sessions only. So I decided that some disaggregation was necessary. Thus an afternoon clinic was started for gynaecological troubles which were very common, and another for the lepers. There was little we could do for the latter group at that time except to segregate the patients suffering from the most infectious lepromateus type of the disease. The tuberculoid forms are not very infectious. In fact leprosy is one of the least contagious of the infectious diseases and most people are not liable to contract it because their immune systems usually overcome the mycobacterium. It can now be rendered non-contagious and cured if diagnosed early enough, by a combination of drugs which may have to be continued for prolonged periods, if not for life. We segregated the highly infectious cases and requested their admission to the Western Region Leprosy Colony and Research Centre at Uzuakoli, near Ilesha. Smallpox was dealt with in a small mud-hutted hospital two miles outside the town where immunised nurses looked after the patients and the sanitary staff vaccinated as many contacts as they could trace.

I was kept busy in the operating theatre dealing with emergencies and two 'lists' per week. The routine surgery was like that encountered in Bida, without the elephantiasis — hernias, bladder and gallstones and casualty work for injuries from crocodile and bush-cow.

An Administrative Paradox

I have said that the administration was strongly averse to 'bum-punching' as it considered medical officers in government service should not charge money for treating the native population. The medical services' viewpoint on the subject has been clarified above.

Therefore I was surprised one day after I had been in Warri some months to be summoned to the Resident's office and told by him that he was receiving numerous complaints from the various NAs that I was not 'bum-punching' enough. I told him that I was only doing so once a week, much less than my immediate predecessor and possibly less than other medical officers in the past, but that the out-patient clinics at the hospital were full to overflowing and that very few beds in the wards were ever vacant. What were his own views on the present arrangements? He told me he knew the hospital was busy, a fact that pleased him, but could I not spare some more time going round the province 'bum-punching'? I said that in my view this would not be justifiable and that I would prefer things to stay as they were now organised and so would Dr Joey Walker, the DMS. The matter was never raised again while I served in Warri.

Social Life in Warri

We made many good friends in Warri, especially through our sporting activities. One day, Diana, at the age of fifteen months, decided she would start to walk, a feat she had never achieved until then. She was sitting in her push-chair quietly watching a tennis foursome when she halted the players and ball-boys by getting out of the chair and walking in a tottery fashion all round the perimeter of the court and back to her chair, which she remounted and sat down. The following applause might well have been for Fred Perry!

It was always pleasant, after tennis, golf or snooker, to sit on comfortable chairs on the lawn, between the club building and the jetty sticking out into the creek, in a short gloaming, having a pint of lager, gin and tonic, or a 'coaster' (a long pink gin and soda). By the time Diana was able to walk from chair to chair she had already acquired a taste for lager — people would give her sips from their mugs, in the way small children are spoilt in such surroundings. She was not a hungry child and had the habit of 'pouching' her food in her cheeks, instead of swallowing it. She did the same with the salted peanuts eaten with drinks at the club. One evening, John Hodge, the Superintendent of Police, who had relieved Boycie Peebles, was startled, after he had given Diana her routine swig from his glass-bottomed beer-mug, to finish his drink and find ten peanuts at the bottom.

Food Consumption Studies in Delta Province

The posting to Warri gave me the opportunity to extend my food consumption and clinical studies to include the high forest and fresh water swamp ecological zones and the large area of mangrove swamp which together formed most of the Delta Province. Exactly the same methods were used as in Niger Province at Bida, Kontagora and Zuru. A section of the Western Region Field Medical Unit was trained to measure food consumption and an Ijaw medical orderly from Warri Hospital was put in charge of operations. He rejoiced in the name of Mr John Bull.

The population groups examined were, first, yam and cassava farmers in a village called Illu on the borders of the fresh water swamp and high forest vegetation zones, 5° 40' N and 6° 10' E. Another group was composed of Ijaw fishermen living on an

THE DELTA PROVINCE

island, Soragbemi, in the mangrove swamp, 5° 30' N and 5° 30' E. As a contrast to these subsistence-level farmers and fishermen a group of 'wealthy' male and female traders living in Warri town was chosen for investigation.

I have already explained that there was little seasonal change in food production and consumption in the Delta area. The staple foodstuffs were yams of various species and cassava. Subsistory foodstuffs were maize, plantains, sweet potatoes, cowpeas, lablab and sword beans, and a great variety of wild green leaves and fruit. The fishermen in the mangrove swamps grew a little cassava but bartered their fish to the farmers in the fresh water areas and high forest zone for cassava, yams, sweet potatoes and cowpeas and for logs from which to build their canoes.

Equal numbers of men and women in each group were chosen at random for the food consumption, clinical, biochemical and anthropometric studies, which were carried out on three occasions between April 1949 and April 1950.

I had anticipated trouble with the Ijawa of Soragbemi Island when we asked them to submit to having their food weighed and measured and allow themselves and their womenfolk to participate. They were known to be touchy about their private lives and were also very liable to drink considerable quantities of palm wine obtained from the sap of the Raphia palm as a daily habit. On special days they would drink a spirit distilled from the sap of the Raphia palm, from plantains or from sweet potatoes. This spirit was known to the administration and to the police as 'illicit gin'. There was nothing that could be done to stop its production and consumption at domestic and local level but it was officially banned from sale in the local markets. Every year many miles of copper piping was filched from PWD yards as far away as Lagos for the purpose of making the stills. We found the average daily intake of palm wine to be 250 ml of palm wine among the Urhobo tribe in the fresh water area; they did not drink 'illicit gin'. Among Sorebemi fishermen the mean daily consumption of palm wine throughout the year was over 100 ml/day and of 'illicit gin' 100 ml/day. The latter group tended to drink 'gin' in frenzied bouts to celebrate some special event, after which we would find that the whole population of the small island, from the old men and women down to toddlers, was in various degrees of inebriation.

It was a strain on the members of the Field Medical Unit who were strangers in this area to work in such circumstances, but my faithful Ijaw, John Bull, saw to it that they came to no harm, and they did the weighing and measuring of food satisfactorily and the microscopy work well. On one occasion, when I was spending two nights on the island accompanied by the Provincial Education Officer, we were awakened by a considerable commotion outside our hut and were led by the head man and his senior friends to the middle of a small clearing in the centre of which was a still, bubbling away furiously, and near to it some large pots. The intoxicated natives started to dance round us, insisting that we partake of some neat 'gin' which had a peculiar, but not unpleasant flavour. The pace became more and more furious and John MacKenzie reached the stage of thinking that we were to be boiled alive in the jars when John Bull appeared, the clamour stopped, and he told us we had just been created honorary chiefs of Soragbemi Island. At that moment it was an honour I could well have done without!

The method whereby food and nutrient intakes were compared to a long list of clinical signs and symptoms and to the general appearance, weight, histories of past complaints, biochemical data and prevalence of infectious and infestations again paid dividends in the form of attributing clinical signs to specific nutrient deficiencies. The Illu farmers' and fishermen's diets only provided enough energy to support light activity, judged by the US National Research Council's recommendations (1945) adjusted for body weight, sex and climate. I had first considered that the fishermen had a heavy task, rowing against strong tides, hollowing out their dug-out canoes, from logs obtained in the high forest zone, and pulling in yards of line against the stream. Closer observation showed this was far from the case. He supervised his wives and children in the carpentry of canoe-building, then paddled gently out to his chosen fishing ground, anchored, tied a baited line to one big toe, lay down and went to sleep, come sun, rain or wind. If a fish took his bait he struck by a conditioned reflex action of his foot, woke up and then pulled in maybe fifteen yards of line with his catch.

The Illu farmers also had an easy time growing root crops, their fields being on their own doorsteps or not much more than 200 yards away. Clearing of a new bush was only carried out once every three or four years. The whole process of building yam or cassava heaps or ridges, planting, weeding and harvesting took about thirty days' work in the year. Otherwise their activities were mainly sedentary: weaving, basket-making, repairing primitive huts or gentle dancing and other forms of evening amusement in which they engaged. A family would probably own two or three red-oil palm trees from which they expressed palm oil for sale to UAC and other trading companies and sold the kernels also; they made palm wine from the red-oil palm trees and from Raphia palms. Assuming the energy intake to be equivalent to energy expenditure, provided individual body weights are the same at the beginning and end of a year, it can be inferred that the average daily energy expenditure of the fishermen was 2,190 kcal and that of the farmers 2,150 kcal, their mean body weights being 54.1 kg and 50.5 kg for adult men and women respectively.

The fishermens food supplied 68 g/day of protein from fresh or dried fish, oysters and prawns, another 12 g of protein being derived from cassava, yams and other vegetable sources. The total protein in the Illu farmers' diets was only 46 g/day, but twenty were derived from animal sources, mostly fish but including small amounts from a wide variety of local farms. Included were monkey meat, the giant African snail, oil palm weevils, frog's legs, porcupine, pangolin and the giant Gambian rat. The remaining 26 g of protein in the Illu diet came from yams, cassava, beans and fresh leaves and fruit.

As expected the thiamin and nicotinic acid contents of the Illu and Soragbemi diets were much less than in the northern villages previously studied. Expressed in terms of energy intake only 0.14 mg/1000 kcal/day of thiamin was provided by the fishermen's diet and 0.31 mg/1000 kcal by that of the farmers, compared to NRC recommended allowance of 0.5 mg/1000 kcal for healthy Americans. The intakes of nicotinic acid were not as high in the Delta as in Northern Nigeria but, except for the Illu farmers (4 mg/1000 kcal) the recommended allowance of 5 kg/kcal was met by the fishermen's diet. Clinical pellegra was not observed. In spite of low dietary thiamin frank beri-beri, of either the wet or dry forms, was rarely encountered although neuritis pains, calf tenderness and a degree of emotional instability were clinical features commonly observed.

Dietary riboflavin levels were low and the clinical picture of riboflavin deficiency postulated from the Northern Nigerian data was confirmed and another symptom was added, namely a very irritating dermatosis of the scrotum and external female genitalia. All the signs described — sore lips and tongues, conjunctivitis and this genital dermatosis cleared up completely after the administration of 5 mg synthetic riboflavin daily within a period of two or three weeks.

The traders' diets had three faults: an excess of energy intake over output with resulting weight gains; thiamin was not quite adequate (0.34 mg/1000/kcal/day) and riboflavin did not quite meet requirements, in spite of a small consumption of milk. The signs of riboflavin deficiency were not observed in the traders. The consumption of alcohol was considerable, the mean daily intake throughout the year being as follows — palm wine 120 ml, 'illicit gin' 20 ml, European gin 26 ml, whisky 25 ml, brandy (Spanish) 15 ml, and imported beer 100 ml.

In view of the very heavy rates of infections and infestations to which the populations were exposed it is not surprising that the general appearance was worse than might have been expected from dietary deficiencies alone. Only 70 per cent of the traders were classified as 'good', 26 per cent being 'fair' and 4 per cent 'poor'. The Soragbemi fishermen living at subsistence level were categorised 67 per cent 'good', 30 per cent 'fair' and 3 per cent 'poor', nearly as satisfactory as the wealthy traders of Warri town. The Illu farmers showed the results of their environment and diet more clearly, 38 per cent 'good', 56 per cent 'fair' and 6 per cent 'poor'.

In spite of an apparently very adequate iron intake Hb levels were only 11.5 g/100 ml (traders), 10.6 g/100 ml (fishermen) and 9.8 g/100 ml (farmers). Malignant malaria was holoendemic, yellow fever occurred in small epidemics from time to time as immunity broke down and reinfection from the monkeys, which carried the disease, took place. Viral hepatitis occurred in epidemics. Respiratory diseases, including tuberculosis, were common as were gastro-intestinal troubles such as non-specific dysenteries in children. Amoebic dysentery and liver abscesses were often present. Hookworms were found in 73 per cent of the traders, 96 per cent of the fishermen and 95 per cent of the farmers. Round worms were very common especially in children.

Leprosy and smallpox have been mentioned above. Thus public health and environmental hygiene had to play an important part within any planning for improved nutrition.

It always seemed amazing that the livers of these people could have any physiological capacity left considering the pathological insults which were inflicted on them. Between 56 per cent and 70 per cent of all three groups showed urobilinogenuria. Up to 19 per cent of all livers were enlarged.

The Government Chemist in London was kind enough to analyse some of the native millet beers, palm wine and illicit gin for me and found in them a number of different alcohols additional to ethanol, e.g. butyl and methyl alcohols. He was also kind enough to report on the proximate composition and vitamin and mineral content of many of the animal and vegetable foodstuffs which were eaten but not included in any of the food composition tables available to me.

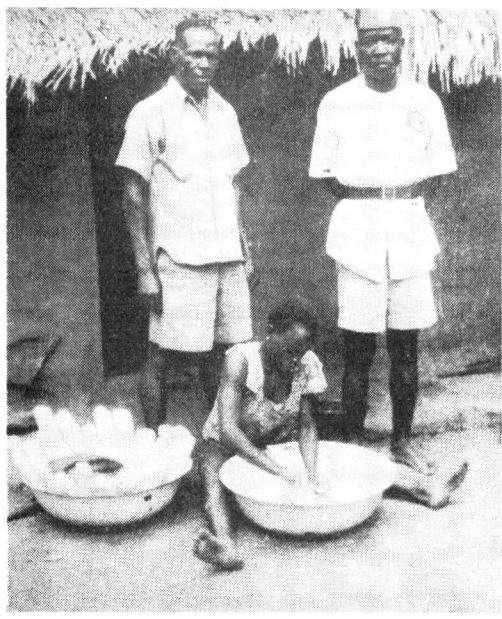

Preparation of gari from peeled cassava root, Ughelli, August 1949.

CHAPTER 8

Return to Warri

Life went on in a routine fashion from June 1949 to June 1950 when the time came for Mary to take Christopher to school at the Edinburgh Academy. He had been entered at birth and should not have come back to Nigeria with us in February 1949. However, for some reason or other, which may well have been the 'Cold War' then being waged in Europe, we had brought him back with us and it was now imperative that he be in the preparatory school boarding house, Mackenzie House, in September 1950, when he would be eight years old.

I saw Mary, C. and Diana off from Sapele in the SS *Salagar,* an Elder Dempster ship carrying twelve passengers as well as cargo. Captain Lewis was the master. After loading logs at Sapele the *Salagar* lay off Lagos for a week or so loading cocoa. Mary saw Dick Greswell and his wife Jean, Ron Berriff and other Lagos friends. Then they stopped at Takoradi (Gold Coast), Las Palmas for fuel, and nearly put into a Spanish port to land a lady passenger believed to have appendicitis. Mary tells me nearly all the passengers went down with tummy trouble at one point, for which malady Captain Lewis favoured a hefty dose of castor oil as a cure, and apparently it worked.

One day Diana was taken in charge by Captain Lewis after lunch in his cabin, with the door shut to stop her creeping overboard under the rails and into the sea. She had been saved from such a fate twice before, once by Mary and once by Captain Lewis himself. On this occasion after lunch the gallant Captain snoozed off, having secured the door. So Diana went through the drawers of his desk, scattering the contents, and ate a number of his cigarettes — another good opportunity for the administration of castor oil!

Mary and the family stayed with her step-sister (Dick Prothero)

RETURN TO WARRI

in Parkstone until she took C. to Edinburgh in late September 1950 to be left at school. Apparently the parting at Mackenzie House was a sad affair but they both survived it. According to Matron it took C. all of two weeks to find his feet but he then went on to spend ten years at the Academy, moving to Scott House at the age of thirteen and finally passing O-level and A-level exams and eventually obtaining the Scottish Schools Higher Leaving Certificate and passing Certificate A in the Combined Cadet Force, which had been the OTC in may day. He enjoyed the CCF camps as I had done the OTC camps.

I stayed on in Warri until I was relieved by a Maltese Colonial Medical Service doctor, Cauchi by name, after finishing an extra-long two-year tour. While continuing to carry out the routine duties of MO Warri, I started analysing the data obtained from the food consumption and clinical nutrition studies carried out among the Warri traders, Illu farmers and Soragbemi fishermen, and comparing them with the results obtained in Niger Province during my first tour. Meantime I had been made chairman of the Warri Club and, all in all, was feeling and behaving in a very 'end of tourish' manner when eventually I went round to Lagos to board MV *Accra* in February 1951, bound for Liverpool.

We spent leave between seeing Mary's family in Dorset, Edinburgh and Aberdeen. I wrote up the data obtained from Delta Province on food consumption and clinical status, and it was published early in 1952 in the *British Journal of Nutrition*.

Doctoring in Lagos

In June 1951 I was posted to the Creek Hospital in Lagos as physician, Ian Macgregor being the surgeon. This hospital served the British Civil Service officers, senior African civil servants, and the expatriate staff, mostly British, but including French, Italian, Dutch, American, Greek and others of the trading firms which had their headquarters in Lagos. The house that went with this appointment was No. 4 Second Avenue, Ikoyi, a large house with a self-contained spare wing which was useful for guests and visitors.

The two doctors stationed at the Creek Hospital in 1951-52 were the only doctors in Lagos responsible for the senior expatriate and Nigerian staff from the Governor downwards. At that time Sir John Macpherson was Governor; Hugh Foot,

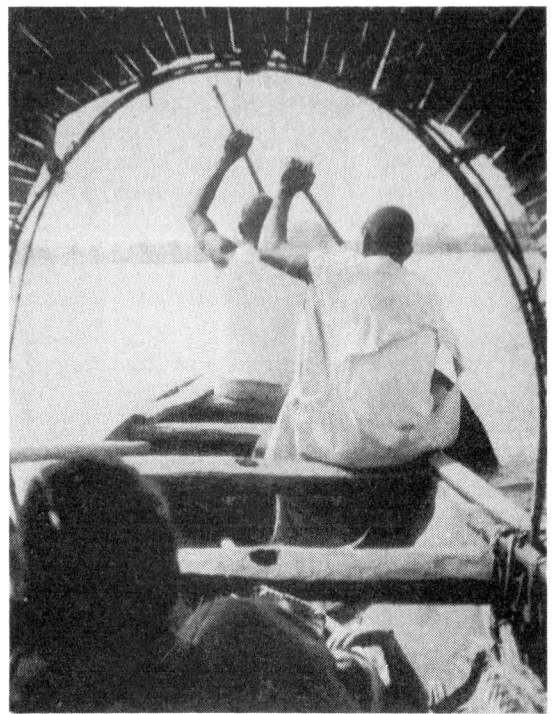

Christmas Eve 1952, in a canoe near the source of the River Niger in Nigeria.

now Lord Caradon, was Chief Secretary; Hugo Marshall was Administrative Secretary, and Clem Pleass, who lived next door to us in No. 6 Second Avenue, was Development Secretary. Clem became the first Lieutenant-Governor of the Eastern Region in 1952 when the title of Chief Commissioner was dropped that year, and Governor of the Eastern Region in 1954 when the regional titles were again changed and the Governor of Nigeria became the Governor-General.

Our friends Dick Greswell and Ron Berriff were still working in the Secretariat in Lagos. Dr Joey Walker had retired and Dr Samuel Manuwa (soon to be Sir Samuel), a Yoruba Nigerian qualified in medicine at the University of Edinburgh, had become the first African in the British Colonial Territories in Africa to become a Director of Medical Services. This was especially important as Nigeria was the largest and most highly populated of all British African colonies.

The staff at the Creek Hospital comprised three and sometimes four European nursing sisters working under the overall supervision of the Matron of Nursing Services at Medical Headquarters. Sister Barbara Earner was the senior sister, very competent technically and a good administrator. The African nurses, with exceptions, were well trained, and the male nurse responsible for the out-patient department, Mr Eda, was technically sound, uniquely tactful and absolutely honest. He had a difficult job pointing out to senior civil servants, expatriate and Nigerian, and to senior members of the oil firms such as Shell, Mobil, Texaco and the other large companies, that precedence for seeing the doctor on duty was strictly *not* influenced by the colour of the patient's skin or his capacity to bribe him. First come first served. He fulfilled this difficult task with great credit to the Medical Services.

We started out-patients at 7 a.m. so that members of the Secretariat could reach their desks by 8 a.m. when that august assembly of administrative officers was expected to start work. It was as good as a play, especially on a Monday morning, to watch certain individuals holding old copies of newspapers or the usual very dated waiting-room magazines in front of their faces for camouflage and nodding the man beside him, also reluctant, towards the surgery door. Ian Macgregor was good at spotting the malingerers. 'The man behind the copy of *Punch*, 1946, I know who you are, and that you have missed two places in the queue. It appears your job in the Secretariat is of little importance, in your opinion, but I now insist that you come here and let me find out if there is anything wrong with you.' The poor man would have to reveal himself, but he was not laughed at, because by this time all those remaining were also merely suffering from hangovers and reluctant to put seat to office chair. The genuinely sick or worried who were keen to work had arrived much earlier and were by now working or on sick leave. Out-patients usually were cleared by 10 a.m. or so and we repaired to Sister Earner's office for a cup of coffee, which was brought by a junior sister.

Ian did all the major surgery, which was not much, and most of the obstetrics and gynaecology. However, one or two husbands

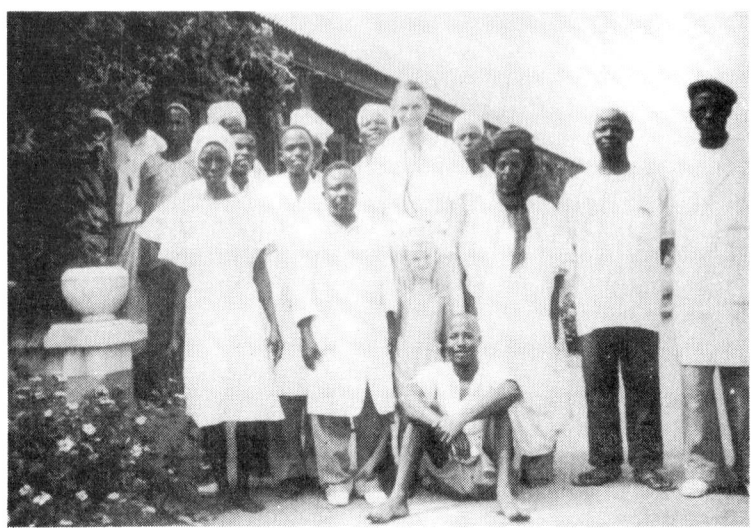

The author with staff of Kaduna Hospital and Christopher.

and wives opted for me to help them and I provided obstetrical care for several young ladies, including a few having their first children in Africa despite advice that they should go home to UK or to their country of origin in Europe or America. Unfortunately for me, Samuel Manuwa, by now DMS, wanted me to look after his wife. She was not a primapara, having had a daughter three years before the pregnancy with which he asked me to help her. Lady Manuwa was a cheerful and healthy Yoruba who had little fear of bearing children, much less than her Edinburgh-trained husband and her Aberdeen/Edinburgh-trained physician acting as an obstetrician. However, all went well and I was able to reach the hospital in time to see Barbara Earner helping Lady Manuwa produce a healthy son at 4 a.m. Why do women so often produce their children at such ungodly hours? I rang Sir Samuel from the Creek and he insisted I go to his house for a drink before he went to see his son. We started to gossip about Edinburgh University and the Royal Infirmary. Eventually I just had time for a bath and a bite of breakfast before reaching the out-patient department at 7 a.m. as usual.

General Practice in Lagos

Working at Creek Hospital was, on the whole, dull, and not the sort of existence which appealed to me. After any operating session and routine rounds I was usually back home for lunch before 2 p.m. followed by a short siesta before going the rounds of the houses to see government servants or members of the trading firms who were either in bed at home or, in the case of non-government people, who had asked for a private domiciliary visit. It was necessary to look after as many patients as possible in their homes because of the limited number of beds in the hospital. Ian Macgregor and John Sorley, from whom I took over as physician at the Creek Hospital, had divided the private, fee-paying, non-government patients into groups based largely upon the firms for which they worked.

This was a financial plum but added a lot of mileage during our evening visiting rounds. I say 'our' because Mary used to drive me round the houses from about 4 p.m. until 6 or 7 p.m. in a new car I had recently purchased, a Wolesley 6/80. This meant she could not play tennis in the evenings but she made up for that by playing with friends in the mornings at the Ikoyi Club.

Research into Effectiveness of Anti-malarial Drugs in European and Other Expatriates

The anti-malarial drugs being taken by European and other expatriates in Lagos in the early 1950s were varied in nature, quantity and periodicity of dosage. There was disagreement between doctors and in the medical press about the best drugs to use for both prophylaxis and for treatment. Therefore I decided to carry out an enquiry into this question, employing the past and present experience of a group of non-natives resident in Nigeria. The group consisted of all the expatriates who reported to my out-patient clinic at the Creek Hospital between 1 November 1951 and 31 March 1952, irrespective of the complaint which brought them to the hospital.

The detailed methodology employed and the results recorded were published in full in the *British Medical Journal* in July 1953. The *BMJ* paper produced some favourable reaction from that section of the medical profession which was experienced in this field. The manufacturers of 'paludrine', the ICI trade name for proguanil, were delighted to know that this was the most effective anti-malarial drug taken at sufficient dosages. A considerable correspondence developed with the Foreign Office and Board of Trade regarding the suppressives being taken by their overseas staff. I am glad to see that in *Practice and Principles of Medicine,* 14th edition, 1984, 200 mg of proguanil daily is still recommended as the best prophylactic for the use in sub-Saharan Africa.

Medical Teaching while Physician at Creek Hospital
The DMS asked me to prepare lectures on gastroenterology to be included in the systematic course given to the students training to be assistant medical officers at the medical school at Yaba. He also wanted me to include a few talks on the work I had done in the Northern and Western Regions which compared food consumption with clinical status and the importance of infections and infestations not only as a public health hazard but in respect of their importance in the actiology of malnutrition. Would I also, please, take the final year medical students on ward rounds in the General Hospital, Lagos, and point out the clinical manifestations of general under-nutrition and malnutrition, the signs of specific nutrient deficiencies such as ariboflinosis, pellegra, scurvy, rickets, iron deficiencies and so on? It was fun to take groups of students round wards again.

I was also appointed co-examiner in medicine at the University of Ibadan, where I first met Derrick Jelliffe, the Professor of Medicine, later to become a world-renowned 'nutritionist'. He and his wife, Patrice, were already working together on problems of nutrition in infants and young children and I enjoyed my visits to Ibadan University Medical School very much. Jelliffe was the second Professor of Medicine in Ibadan. The first, who had founded the Faculty, was an ex-colleague of mine, Sandy Brown from Edinburgh University.

A Federal Approach to Food and Nutrition
While working in the Creek Hospital I gave some thought to the expansion of research work at the Federal Nigerian level along the lines I had started in Niger Province in the Northern Region and Delta Province in the Western Region. It would be a great help to Agriculture, Forestry and Fisheries development programmes if a wider knowledge of the relationship between food production, food consumption and health in the different

ecological zones of the whole country was available. The Northern Regional Nutrition Committee had become active again since my tour in Niger Province but the Eastern and Western Regions, whilst having such bosies on paper, never met. Hence I pressed the DMS (Sir Samuel Manuwa) and my friends in the Secretariat, particularly Frank Williams, responsible for Finance, and Tom Scrivenor from the personnel point of view, to consider the possibility of setting up a Federal Food and Nutrition Unit which would be responsible for collecting the information needed to prepare what I then called a 'food and nutrition' map covering the whole of the territory. I also lobbied the two Development Secretaries who succeeded each other while I was physician at the Creek Hospital, namely Clem Pleass and Ralph Grey. I was extremely well supported by the Federal Chief Conservator of Forests, Don Rosevear, who had first pointed out to me the importance of such work in the development context.

I had proposed a minimum staff establishment for such a Federal Medical Nutrition Unit. It would include one biochemist, one African assistant medical officer qualified from Yaba, one laboratory technician trained in biochemistry, one clerk/stenographer, two laboratory attendants and one driver. I listed what I considered then to be a minimum of laboratory equipment plus one station-wagon, one two-ton lorry and one 15-cwt. truck.

For some months there was absolutely no reaction to my proposal. Then, quite out of the blue, two proposals reached me. The first was by telephone from the Federal Financial Secretary (Frank Williams) to tell me that the Federal Development Committee had decided in principle to include a Federal Nutrition Unit on the establishment starting in the financial year 1953/54; details of finances and personnel would have to be worked out later. The second was that WHO had been authorised to ask the Nigerian government if I would be available to be granted a Nutrition Fellowship for six-nine months starting in 1952: it was, by now, January 1952. The DMS immediately accepted the fellowship on my behalf and together we discussed likely dates. I was, rather naturally, keen to take up the fellowship as soon as possible so that I could be back in Nigeria long before April 1953 when the Federal Nutrition Unit would come into being, in fact and not only on paper. Eventually Sir Samuel decided I should start the fellowship in May 1952, but go on leave in April, have

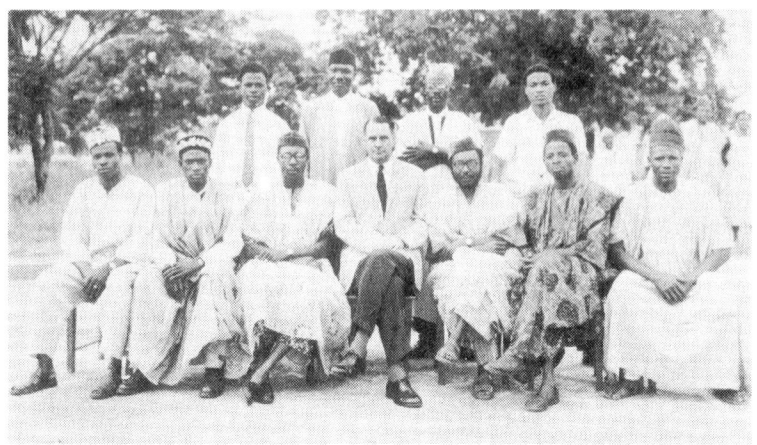

With nutrition unit, Kaduna.

three weeks' leave and ask my friends in Edinburgh how best I should use the WHO grant.

We duly arrived in the UK and stayed in Edinburgh while I discussed with Peter Meiklejohn, an old friend from the University, how best to use my fellowship. He knew the most important nutritionists in the USA. With Reg Passmore, another Edinburgh friend, I discussed how I could help in a study of the energy expenditure of coal miners in Fife, for which he was making his preparations. This study was being sponsored by the Medical Research Council of the Privy Council (MRC) to find out if there was still justification for the additional food rations which, in 1952, miners received over and above those of the population in general. Prof. Stanley Davidson gave me good advice about physicians in the UK who were interested in questions of food and nutrition, a few of whom had worked in tropical countries.

From June to August 1952 I toured the United Kingdom to meet professionals in the field of nutrition, some of who I had met before and some I knew only from their work.

I visited Professor B. S. Platt at London University and we discussed thiamin deficiency and beri-beri and then Dr Hugh Sinclair, working at the Churchill Hospital in Oxford, where we tried to resolve the difference between 'under-nutrition' and 'famine'. At the Postgraduate Hospital in Hammersmith Professor

John McMichael helped me to update my knowledge of clinical medicine and Dr E. J. King gave me advice on the best methods of determining levels of haemoglobin plasma protein in blood and carrying out liver function tests in the field. After meeting several colleagues in Cambridge I drove to Birmingham and learnt a lot from Professor Alistair Fraser about his work with infants.

I returned to Edinburgh for important discussions with Peter Meiklejohn concerning those nutritionists in the USA I should try to meet. WHO wanted to know as soon as possible who I would propose for the information of their Washington office which was responsible for making arrangements for appointments and travel within the country.

Having sent this information to WHO it was time to prepare for the study on the coal miners in the 'Kingdom of Fife' called for by the MRC Committee under the chairmanship of Professor R. C. Garry of Glasgow University, as a part of the national investigation into problems of diet and energy requirements. This part of the overall study, carried out under the immediate supervision of Reg Passmore, was designed to measure the energy expenditure and food consumption of underground miners and colliery clerks for twenty-four hours a day over a period of one week in July 1952. The colliery chosen was the Wellesley at Buckhaven, Fife.

The main results of this study showed that the daily expenditure of the underground miners was understandably greater than that of the clerks. The study was reported in full to HM Stationery Office Medical Research Council, spec. report series No. 289 (1955).

Participation in this survey at the coal face and in the laboratory gave me good experience to improve my knowledge of methods for the measurement of food consumption, energy expenditure and gas analysis which was to be useful in my future work in Nigeria.

My time in the United States was as rewarding as the study period in Britain though the travel was considerably more taxing. I visited Maryland, N. Carolina, Alabama, Tennessee, Ohio, Minnesota, Illinois and travelled down the East Coast from Boston to Washington until, in January 1953, it was time to return to Liverpool and board ship for Lagos, with Mary and Diana.

CHAPTER 9

Back to Kaduna

Political advances had taken place since I was last in N. Nigeria. The Chief Commissioner had now become Lieutenant-Governor, who was by then Sir Bryan Sharwood-Smith, my Resident at Minna in Niger Province when I was first posted to Nigeria. Ministers had been appointed to be in charge of the different departments, e.g. health, education and agriculture, each ministry having a permanent secretary drawn from the ranks of administrative officers. The Premier of Northern Nigeria was the Sardauna of Sokoto, and my old friend, Makaman Bida, was Minister of Education. Before I left the country in 1960 this political advance had continued and each region became, to all intents and purposes, autonomous with its own Governor, Ministries and Houses of Assembly. Lagos was the federal capital with a Governor-General presiding over a House of Representatives which reflected, more or less, the numbers of the populations in each of these regions. The House of Representatives was responsible overall for foreign affairs, defence and police. After a short leave I went to Kaduna to take up the post of Senior Medical Officer in March 1953. In fact Kaduna was an artificial town which had grown up around Lord Lugard's administration when he moved his HQ northwards from Zunguru, about 1914. I also looked after Sir Bryan Sharwood-Smith and his family at Government Lodge and the Sardauna at his own house.

'Kwashiorkor' or Energy Protein Malnutrition and Liver Diseases
In the General Hospital we had large numbers of patients suffering from enlargement and deformities of the liver, both in male and female adults and in the one to six-year-old group of toddlers. The admissions from the latter group were so high that it became necessary to open a small ward of ten beds for

these children only, suffering from 'kwashiorkor', or protein malnutrition as the clinical syndrome was then described, from a word in the language of the Gold Coast first brought into use by Cicely Williams in 1933, in her view meaning 'the disease the child gets when the next baby is born'. It has also been taken to mean 'red child' as the hair may be mispigmented a somewhat pale reddish tinge. Both these efforts to translate the word 'kwashiorkor' have been heatedly denied by Dr Fred Sai who was born on the Gold Coast. He considered the word to mean the sickness often suffered by young Gold Coast children of the toddler age group.

It must be made quite clear that most of the children suffering from this syndrome were admitted from families of the lower income groups living in the shanty areas close to, or inside, the township of Kaduna and that this high hospital incidence of kwashiorkor was not reflected in the rural villages where I had previously worked which were occupied by farmers living at true subsistence levels. In such villages the prevalence of kwashiorkor was not high in the toddler age group, being 1.4 per cent of all children in that group (0-5 years) and 0.78 per cent in the age group 6-9 years in the grain-eating areas of Northern Nigeria and 3.6 per cent and 1.8 per cent in the root-eating areas of Southern Nigeria (Nicol, B.J.N., 1959, 13, 307). These prevalences were not significantly different.

Kwashiorkor in Africa (Brock and Autret, WHO Monograph Series No. 8) was based on visits between mid-October to mid-December 1950, paid by these authors to ten English and French-speaking colonies where data was gathered from the DMS, hospital assistants, health visitors, missionaries, school teachers and at dispensaries. By their own admission, 'time did not allow extensive visits to rural areas but a certain number of these *accessible to the main centre* (my italics) were visited'. Their report was widely circulated and one of their conclusions was given wide recognition: 'It might be no exaggeration to say that in many parts of Central Africa the majority of the children in the second year of life suffer from kwashiorkor. Unfortunately, final judgement on this point must be reserved until the true significance of dyspigmentation (of the hair and skin) is understood.' They believed that the syndrome is due to the deficiency in the diet of some factor or factors which are originally supplied by foods containing animal protein or certain of the vegetable proteins of higher biological value. The same criticism, that surveys were only conducted in and around hospital centres, can be levelled at the reports by Autret and Behar, *Kwashiorkor and its Prevention in Central America* (FAO Nutrition Study No. 13, 1954), and *Protein Malnutrition in Brazil* (Waterlow and Vergars, FAO Nutrition Study No. 14, 1956) and by Collis in *A Doctor's Nigeria* (Secker and Warburg, London, 1960).

Jumping the gun by some years my own studies in whole communities of subsistence farmers living in the bush in North and South Nigeria up to 1960, and this group was believed by the Department of Statistics to comprise 80 per cent of the country's population, indicated the following major factors in the aetiology of kwashiorkor in order of frequency:

(a) *Breast failure.* 29 per cent most often due to breast abscesses.
(b) *Malnutrition of the mother.* 24 per cent, particularly during times of food shortage.
(c) *Maternal infections or infestations.* 23 per cent, such as pneumonia, dysentery, malaria and amoebiasis, schistosomiasis or ankylosomiasis leading to severe anaemia.
(d) *Dysentery.* 17 per cent occurring in the child.
(e) *Subsequent pregnancy.* 5 per cent. This low figure is due to the fact that sexual intercourse normally does not take place during lactation, a very wise traditional habit practised by all the people living in the rural areas at subsistence level.
(f) *Undetermined.* 2 per cent.

(The above figures were presented in a lecture given to fourth year medical students of Cornell University in 1961 in the UN Building in New York, and have not been published elsewhere.)

But it was not only the prevalence of 'protein malnutrition' and enlarged livers in infants and toddlers which fuelled my interest in the aetiology and pathology of liver disease at the time I was SMO Kaduna. I had found, during my surveys in Niger Province that 17.7 per cent of adults had clinical manifestation of hepatic abnormality and/or a previous history of jaundice, the equivalent figure from the people studied in Delta Province being 15.7 per cent. Therefore I decided to start a systematic histological examination of the livers of all age groups using either needle biopsy as practised by Waterlow in Jamaica or by taking small sections of liver tissue on every case which had required surgical intervention involving laparatory (opening of the abdominal cavity).

I sent over one hundred liver sections so obtained to Professor John MacMichael at the Postgraduate Hospital in London. He kindly made arrangements for them to be examined in the Pathology Department of the Westminster Hospital where an electron microscope was available. I had hoped to be able to correlate the food consumption of the patients with the histological pictures. Unfortunately the pathologists at the Westminster Hospital found such a high proportion of the liver sections to show infestation with, e.g. schistosome eggs, amoebae in both the vegetative and cystic forms, malaria parasites in the red cells in both portal arteries and hepatic veins, ankylostome larvae, and trypanosomes in the portal tracts that it was impossible to say which came first, the infestations or the possibility of pathological change caused by any nutrient deficiency.

Nevertheless the whole of the period of four months spent on the investigation of the relationship between nutrient intake and pathological changes in the liver was of interest, even if it only showed the damage done by infestations to the structure and function of the liver and gave little information about the effects of specific nutrient deficiencies, such as lack of dietary protein or of labile methyl groups.

While SMO at Kaduna I was able to start the work of the Federal Nutrition Unit in premises belonging to the West African Institute for Trypansomiasis Research. By a reciprocal agreement FNU and WAITR would use any equipment which might save duplication of costs. These instructions were made as a gentlemen's agreement and no official papers required signing or ratification by the Chief Medical Adviser to the Federal Government in lagos. The system worked without any trouble until I left the FNU and Nigeria in 1960 upon the attainment by the territory of full federal independence.

The vagaries of chance here again helped greatly and made it possible to start and expand the work of the FNU much more quickly than would otherwise have been possible. Early in 1953 the Colonial Medical Research Committee decided to close down the Hot Climate Physiological Research Unit which had been entirely financed by Colonial Development and Welfare Funds, and established at Oshodi, on the mainland near Lagos

WIND OF CHANCE

Island. The Director, Dr W. S. S. Ladell, was transferred to the top secret UK Government Research Laboratory at Porton in England. However, his biochemist, Mr Peter G. Phillips, and most of the African technical staff who had worked with him, would have been jobless if the FNU had not started work in April 1953. Ladell and Phillips had been working on the energy expenditure of agricultural workers in Western Nigeria; on nitrogen balance in Nigerians; on groundnut flour as a dietary protein source in local diets, and on the energy and nutrient composition of Nigerian foodstuffs. It seemed too good to be true that I should be able to obtain the services of an English biochemist and well-trained African laboratory technicians, already working in the field of food composition and nutrition, plus some secretarial help accustomed to the technical jargon. Sir Samuel Manuwa, by now the Chief Medical Adviser to the Federal Government, was delighted to agree to the transfer of Phillips and those of his technicians he would like to bring with him to the FNU in Kaduna, provided the FNU budget would cover their salaries. In the end Peter Phillips, his chief laboratory technician, Mr Cshinyemi, and his chief clerk, Mr Aggobokhaevbo, came north to Kaduna, bringing an assortment of very useful laboratory equipment with them.

I had to decide what transport would be needed to carry our field staff and mobile laboratory to whose areas where the food consumption, clinical and biochemical surveys would be carried out in the different ecological zones. We eventually settled for one three-ton lorry, fitted with a kerosene burning refrigerator, to carry all our equipment, and a 30-cwt. lorry for the staff and their bedding and tents, plus a 15-cwt. truck for bits and pieces. I had by this time bought a five-seater Chevrolet with a large boot, a pale cream roof and strangely shimmering brown-coloured body, known as 'Connie'. She lasted for five years running mainly on corrugated laterite roads, covering 130,000 miles before she became too costly to run and maintain. We were all very fond of her and sorry to exchange her for a Peugeot 403 station-wagon ('Pip') for the last two years of my time in Nigeria. I recruited my old friend and assistant from Bida and Kontagora days, Mallam Abubakar Zukogi Bida, to assist me in the future work on food consumption, at which he had proved himself to be painstaking and adept.

Programme of Work for Federal Nutrition Unit

As already indicated, the work which had to be considered of highest priority was to develop a food consumption map covering the different ecological zones of Nigeria and to relate this food consumption, expressed in terms of energy and nutrients, with the various populations' health determined by detailed clinical, anthropometric and biochemical studies. The collection of such data would provide base-lines from which to advise the government in developing agricultural, forestry and fisheries development policies and for measurement of the future development of the population's state of health. Answers to questions relating food consumption to fertility and demography were requested by the Federal Department of Statistics and we did our best to obtain such data. This department told me that over 80 per cent of the Nigerian peoples were not involved in a cash economy so it was decided that this group of farmers, cattle herdsmen or fishermen should be the first target for the compilation of our map. The following stringent criteria were applied in selecting the sample populations. Each collection of compounds, hamlet or village, should be situated at least fifty miles from a town of 5,000 or more inhabitants and at least fifteen miles from a main road or railway. *All* the occupants of the community being studied would be examined clinically and biochemically and for parasites. The food consumption of every third compound would be measured by the methods we had developed in Niger and Delta Provinces. The Field Medical Unit of the different regions under the supervision of Mallam Abubakar would be responsible for measuring food consumption and infestation rates. A course involving practical field trials in villages near Kaduna and in the Sabon Gari was organised for the medical units of the Northern and Eastern Regions.

Full details of the methods followed to ascertain food consumption, biochemical and anthropometric data and the prevalence of infections and infestations are given in *British Journal of Nutrition*, (1959), *13*, 293 and 307.

The food consumption surveys should also try to cover different tribal groups in the different ecological zones. Already in Delta and Niger Provinces data had been obtained on adult men and women of the following tribes: the animist Ijawa in the mangrove swamps and Isoko on the edge of the fresh-water swamps and rain forest; the Muslim and pagan Nupe in the southern part and the pagan Gwari and Muslim Fulani in the northern part of the Guinea Savannah zone, and the pagan Dakakerri in the southern regions of the Sudan Savannah. Information was still needed from Sahel Savannah in the north-eastern limits of Nigeria; from somewhere in the area where the Guinea Savannah borders upon the Sudan Savannah; from the High Plateau; from the rain forest; and from the derived savannah.

In the end villages and hamlets meeting our criteria were selected; in the far south-west corner of the country, Tangaza in Sokoto Province where the population was Muslim Fulani and the country was at the northern limit of the Sudan Savannah; in the far north-west, Jarawaji in Sahel Savannah on the shores of Lake Chad, peopled by the Muslim Kanuri and Shuwa Arabs; Bunga on the edge of Sudan and Guinea Savannah, where the people were Hausa-speaking Muslim Fulani; Langai on the High Plateau sixty miles from Jos off the road between Panyam and Pankshin, occupied by pagans of the Kanam tribe; in the derived savannah on the western frontier of Nigeria with Dahomey, the small village of Okuta with a population of mixed pagan, Muslim and Christian Yorubas; and in the rain forest near the Nigeria/South Cameroon boundary a hamlet called Mbanege, near Obudu in Ogojo Province, where the people were of the pagan Boki clan.

The approximate distance, as the crow flies, from Kaduna to Tangaza was 480 miles, to Bunga 250 miles, to Langai 260 miles, to Obudu 450 miles and to Bero-Okuta 270 miles. With no exception in those days the main roads we had to use were not surfaced and were formed of laterite, more or less corrugated by the traffic they carried. In the dry season any vehicle raised a cloud of red, penetrating dust filling one's hair and clothes; in the rainy season many parts of the roads became muddy quagmires. Only people who have often travelled long distances on such roads can understand what I am talking about.

We started the surveys at the end of 1953 and did not finish them until the end of 1957. I have enormous admiration for the enthusiasm which was maintained over these four years by the Regional Field Medical Units, both the food consumption enumerators and the microscopists, the driver-mechanics and the drivers, and for the work of Mallam Abubakar Zukogi Bida who, in his quiet determined way, very tactfully organised the studies of food consumption.

In the early days of the food consumption, clinical and biochemical surveys the laboratory staff of the FNU in Kaduna was cutting its teeth on determining the energy value, moisture content and proximate composition of the staple foods we found to be consumed. The same was done for other foods which made major contributions to the energy and nutrient compositions of the diets. I hoped that our surveys in Nigeria would allow a comparison to be made between the measured energy and nutrient intake recommended by the US National Research Council and by FAO or allowances thus showing where deficiencies occurred in the different age groups of the populations studied. Gaps between recommended allowances and intake could thus be translated into adjustments needed to food crop production and to the consumption of foodstuffs growing wild, very often products of trees. These observations would give the agriculture, forestry and fisheries departments guidelines for planning production strategies on a nutritional basis. Education of senior personnel in these departments on the relationship between food production, food consumption and health would be needed to provide bases for any overall changes I might be able to recommend. A course was organised for representatives of these departments from all these regions in Kaduna in 1954. The Department of Information should also play a part and was included in the course. Eventually I gave three talks on the Lagos nationwide radio which were published as an illustrated manual for general information.

Touring in the Survey Areas

Six areas were involved and three visits of at least ten days duration per annum to each of them at the correct time of year took a considerable amount of organisation not only of the FNU but also of the Field Medical Units. Apart from the first visit, during which I reconnoitred the area and Mallam Abubakar and I explained the reasons for our presence and persuaded the headman to gain the co-operation of his people, not always an easy task, I was accompanied by Mary, and Diana and Christopher if they were on school holidays. We were often the first white people to be seen in these remote areas and the local people were fascinated by our children and what they wore, especially their small shoes which I insisted they wore whenever out of bed.

The team we took from the FNU in Kaduna consisted only of Mallam Abubakar, a driver mechanic who drove the three-tonner, and drivers for the 30-cwt. and 15-cwt. trucks. None of our survey sites had a dispensary or a dressing station so I picked up a female nurse or midwife from the nearest place available. She helped me with the collection of urinary and faecal samples which had to be collected from women.

In addition to the laboratory equipment I had to take, we carried the basic materials and medicines for running an out-patient clinic. This was an essential part of all surveys and was one of the activities which encouraged the people to participate in the food consumption, clinical, anthropometric and biochemical procedures inflicted on them. Every evening about 6 p.m. I held a clinic which was always very well attended and was similar in many ways to the 'medical camps' which Bill Berry had introduced to Nyasaland before and during the Second World War. We also had to take with us the apparatus for measuring weights and heights; a yard-arm balance and a fixed vertical pole with head arm and a board for small children, also the Longworth skin-fold thickness calipers. The kerosene-operated refrigerator was essential for carrying vaccines, chemical re-agents and other heat-perishable substances.

In the car with us we always carried not one spare tyre but two, jerry cans of petrol, two jerry cans of unfiltered water, a water filter and two spare fan belts. Our own 'kitchen' consisted of two primus stoves, two pressure cookers, some pots and pans, plates and camp cutlery. Pressure cookers use much less filtered and boiled water than open pans and one can be used for vegetables and the other for a bush chicken or game bird such as duck, teal or lesser bustard if and when shot. Mary used the primus stoves and pressure cookers while Bernard prepared the food. My old 16-bore shotgun from pre-war days and a 12-bore I had 'picked up' in Germany in 1945 were very useful and cartridges were not hard to come by, even if a little expensive.

The Northern and Eastern Regional Field Medical Units were well accustomed to bush-whacking and looked after themselves very well. Their normal work consisted of mapping the prevalence of infestations and infections such as malaria, schistomiasis and so on. One of their main functions was to spot the beginnings of epidemics of cerebrospinal meningitis (CSM), measles, whooping cough or the like, or to be sent to areas where epidemics had broken out in order to treat cases and contacts in an effort to contain such infectious diseases. Fortunately, during our surveys, we never ran into such an epidemic.

The long hours spent on the laterite roads, through every sort of vegetation from this rain forest to Sahel savannah, without much in the way of game to observe except monkeys of various species, baboons and a few herds of antelope, and occasional lion and elephant were boring for Diana who was six years when we started the surveys. She sat on a special seat we had rigged up between the driver and passenger seats in the front of 'Connie'. When we were travelling *en famille* I tried to restrict the distance we covered daily to 200-250 miles. We could stay at 'catering' rest houses where we had beds and had dinner and breakfast, thus giving our boys a rest. For instance on a journey to Lake Chad from Kaduna, when travelling with Mary and Diana, we would stop at the famous Hill Station in Jos, more of a small hotel with separate chalets. That was 120 miles, then Jos to Potiskum catering rest house was 210 miles. Potiskum to Maiduguri catering rest house (120 miles) and then from Maiduguri up to the mud rest house in Jarawaji (100 miles) on the bank of Lake Chad near the mouth of the river Ngadda which was our survey village. The last ten miles to the village from Ngala on the Maiduguri-Fort Lamy road had to be driven through trackless Sahel thorn scrub using a compass to maintain a due north direction until we hit the lake shore or the river. It was difficult going for the three-ton lorry but the ground was firm even in the short wet season.

Information obtained from the 1954/57 Nigerian
Food and Nutrition Surveys

It took a long time to analyse all the data which had been collected from the seven different areas. Eventually two papers were published in the *British Journal of Nutrition*, 1959, 13, giving the information required. The papers were entitled 'The Calorie Requirements of Nigerian Peasant Farmers' and 'The Protein Requirements of Nigerian Peasant Farmers'.

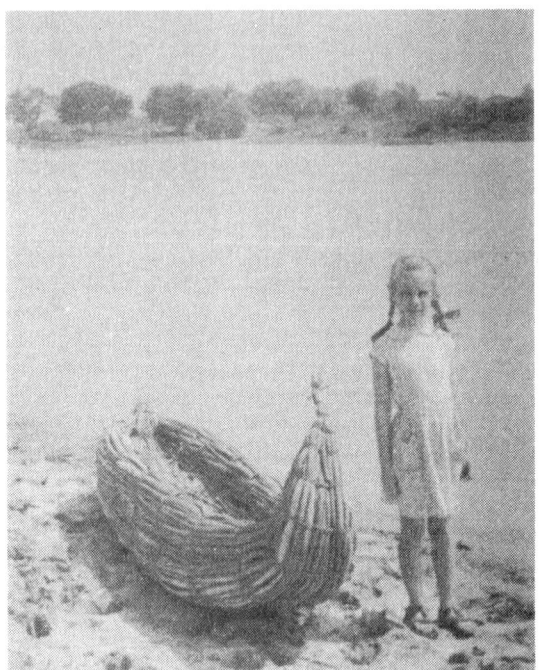

Diana with straw canoe near Lake Chad.

We had learned a great deal about the energy expenditure, and hence requirements, of rural Nigerian farmers and cattle herdsmen and those of their wives and children. We had also quantified to some extent the effects of crop failures upon the activities of cereal and root crop farmers.

In regard to protein requirements we had found that the FAO (1957) Safe Practical Allowances were too high when applied to the diets consumed by subsistence farmers relying either on cereals or roots as their major crops and staple foodstuffs. This conclusion applied to people who were not 'healthy' in the FAO sense of the word but to people who were living in areas where Plasmodium falsiparum malaria was holoendemic, where tuberculosis, leprosy and other infections were common, and where the prevalence of intestinal and other parasites, particularly in children, was very high.

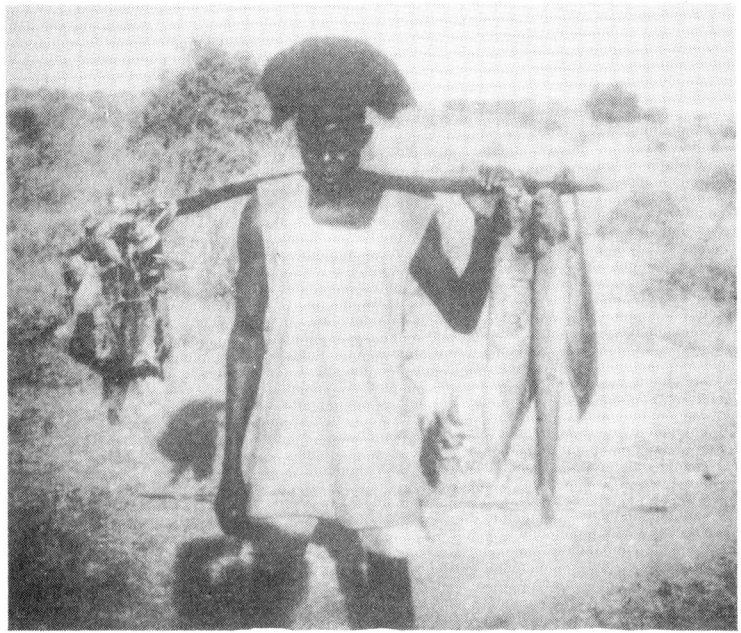

A catch of Lake Chad fish (large ones are Heterotis).

The surveys showed that signs of vitamin deficiencies were rare except for those attributable to lack of vitamin A (retinol) in the northern areas, and of riboflavin in places where milk was not a regular item of diet. The very high concentration of vitamin C (ascorbic acid) found in the dry white powdery pulp surrounding the seeds of the baobab fruit was found to be a major factor in preventing the development of scurvy in the Sahel and Sudan savannah areas (Nature (1957), *180*, p. 287).

The overall picture of the nutritional status of the Nigerian population, and of their food consumption, was not as bad as that reported from the countries further north into the Sahara desert or westward in the northern French Cameroons and the Southern Sudan. The potential for increased quantity of food existed provided good attention was paid to health, agricultural and forestry departments planning along lines suggested by the nutritional findings.

It may be argued that the time spent by the Field Medical Units' staff and by the Federal Nutrition Unit was excessive and costly, but the possibilities and financing were available. All that was needed to conduct the surveys satisfactorily was administration and hard work which was given unstintingly by those involved, and I believe that the results were valuable. Nowadays, when reading or reviewing papers on food consumption by twenty-four-hour 'recall' methods or only a few days of measured food intake, often divorced from clinical features or anthropometric measurements, one feels that the present limitations of funds or staff, and various means of cutting corners, do not result in information which is truly representative of the facts.

Effects of Food and Nutrition Surveys on Planning

During the whole of my service in Nigeria, whether as MO of the Bida medical area, while in Lagos as physician at the Creek Hospital, or adviser on nutrition to the Federal Government, I had kept in close touch with the administration and the departments of health, agriculture, forestry, fisheries and education. Almost without exception the directors of technical departments, or ministries as they became with advancement towards independence, both at federal and regional level, listened to my proposals to include measures designed to modify food crop production and encourage conservation of trees and forests which produced important food items using professional, school and adult education programmes as media for spreading the necessary information.

A factor which was realised by 1954 to be of great importance regarding food supplies was the increasing numbers of the population. The Department of Statistics had asked me if, through our surveys, the FNU could obtain information on the rate of this increase in the rural areas. Data for the increase of the urban and peri-urban population was not difficult to measure, but the statisticians had little accurate knowledge of the demographical situation in the remote rural areas which, as they reconfirmed to me, accounted for what they believed to be over 80 per cent of the total national figures. Therefore the FNU, with the help of the Field Medical Units, assumed an extra function. This required very careful questioning of every female included in the surveys who had reached the *menarche*, and cross-checking with husbands, parents and neighbours, the number of times they had been married; the number, sex and age of children they had produced now alive and the number and sex of any who had died. The ages of the children were determined using the statements of parents and neighbours, state of dentition, general appearance, weight and height. The ages of adults was estimated, as usual, by references to parents and neighbours and to well-known local or world events. From the information so collected the reproductive roots, crude animal birth rate, fertility and sterility rates, infant mortality rates and the mortality rate in the age group 1-4 years were calculated. The data indicated an increase in the rural areas of approximately 2 per cent per annum, compatible with the conclusions drawn by the Department of Statistics from the census figures of 1931 and 1952. Full details were published in the *West African Medical Journal,* February 1959. Important findings were that in both the grain and the root areas, the crude annual birth rate (number of births per annum per 1,000 of the population) was 57; the fertility rate (number of births per annum per 1,000 women of child-bearing age, 15-45 years) was 200 and the sterility rate (number of women per 1,000 women 18 years of age and over, married a minimum of three years) was 65, the infant mortality rate (number of infants per 1,000 live births dying below the age of one year) was 270 and the mortality of toddlers dying between one year and the end of the fourth year was 110 per 1,000 live births. Thus the infant and toddlers' mortality rate from live birth to the end of the fourth year amounted to 380/1,000. Yet in spite of these high sterility rates the rural population was increasing at a rate of 2 per cent per annum compound. There was no demonstrable relationship between the energy and nutritive values of diets and reproductive performance.

Such information raised ethical problems. Improving the public health by efficient environmental hygiene and better medical care in dispensaries and hospitals, coupled with widespread successful immunising programmes such as those being practised by Dr David Morley at Ilesha, would increase birth rates, reduce the 0-4 years mortality rate and undoubtedly result in a faster rate of population growth. Could food production within Nigeria keep pace with such a rate of increase so that sufficient dietary energy could be provided and the patterns of nutrient intakes be improved? The Federal Government did not want to start importing large quantities of foodstuffs from overseas. The only answer to this situation seemed to be the introduction of acceptable methods of birth control. But most Nigerian families, particularly in the rural areas at subsistence economy level, considered large families as their life insurance premium, particularly as nearly half of those live-born died before attaining the age of five years, a mortality rate which might be reduced by successful public health and curative medical methods. How, then, were these people to be persuaded to accept birth control? The answer is that they were not so persuaded as will be discussed later.

Planning for Food Production and Consumption
The results of the surveys regarding energy and nutrient intakes in the different ecological zones compared to the requirements proposed by FAO gave the FNU sufficient information to draw up a plan in very general terms for agricultural, forestry, fisheries and educational activities. When the Federal Director-General of Agriculture asked me to give him a short statement on how planning should proceed I told him 'more fruit and vegetables north of the Niger-Benue line and south of that line replace the production and consumption of roots by rice grown in Nigeria and parboiled, not polished'. The problem then arose — how was this very simplified concept of agricultural production to be implemented?

Since the occupation of Kano by Lord Lugard in 1903, if not before, some of the citizens had made a small income by selling the night-soil collected and carefully composted to the farmers in the surrounding rural areas. They grew vegetables of various sorts, both indigenous such as amaranths and okra, and exotic imported from UK such as cabbages, lettuces and cauliflowers, on the fadamas (floodplains of the small streams and marshland) which surrounded the city. One of the features of the roads leading into Kano from all directions was the number of donkeys with twin panniers containing compost leaving the city and making for the farms. As far as I can remember the cost to the farmer in about 1950 was 4d (four pence) for two pannier load. This revenue went towards the Kano NA public health budget. Although most of the consumers of these vegetables were expatriates who paid the farmers well for them, some education

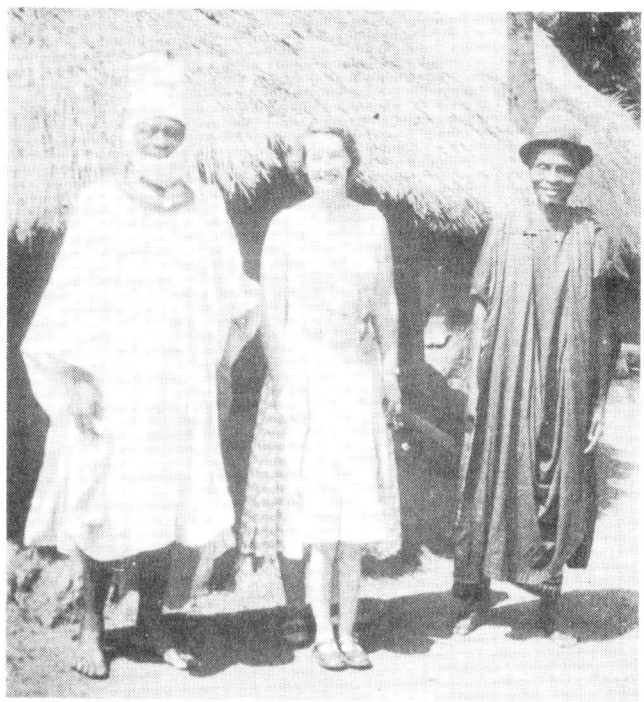

The author's wife and daughter.

about the importance to health of eating such foodstuffs had been impressed upon the local population by Dr W. W. McCulloch during the 1920s and 1930s. He it was who insisted, and rightly so, that all such vegetables eaten by European civil servants and other expatriates, should be carefully washed in a solution of potassium permanganate prepared with filtered and boiled water. This was an essential practice followed by nearly all 'white faces' when eating uncooked green or other vegetables throughout the country. In Bida my predecessor, Dr Macnamara, had started to compost the night soil from the Government Reservation for use as fertiliser in vegetable gardens and from the town of Bida for the use of the surrounding farmers.

In the small compound of the MO's house in Bida we grew some of our own vegetables, mostly indigenous amaranths (A-caudatus) and climbing spinach (Basella alba). We also planted some citrus fruit and cashew nuts (Aracardium occidentale). While our gardener, Bawa, and I were clearing the virgin scrub land on which our new house, 14 Cunliffe Close, was being built, I thought it a good idea to make the compound a demonstration of what could be grown in the way of fruit and vegetables. The Director of Agriculture, Northern Region (Phil Chambers), who was enthusiastic about the idea of increasing the cultivation of those foodstuffs throughout the region, sent us lemon and grapefruit seedlings from the regional propagation centre at Shendam, in the lowland area of the southern part of Plateau Province. Diana and I collected a large number of avocado seeds (stones) which we grew in pots on the back verandah of the house before planting them out. Both the citrus seedlings and avocados thrived exceedingly well provided they were watered properly until well established and we finished with one male avocado tree with his eight wives gathered about him. Pawpaw trees (Carica papaya) flourish in the derived and Guinea savannah zones and we had many around our compound, mostly near the kitchen, behind which we grew a prolific guava tree (Psidium guadjava) from a cutting I brought from Kontagora. As a boundary hedge around the compound Bawa planted out seedlings of the pigeon pea (Cajanus cajan) which soon became a thick fence bearing lots of fruit which could be stored if allowed to ripen and dry or could be eaten like green peas, the pods also being edible and tender if picked early enough in their development. Pigeon peas were not popular with the peoples of Nigeria because they did not like the flavour of the immature beans and pods in their soup and the mature dried pea had to be soaked for about twenty-four hours before a prolonged boiling period to soften it for consumption, either whole or pounded. This operation was time consuming and costly in firewood. However, this food provides considerable quantities of riboflavin, thiamine and nicotinic acid, ample energy and good quality protein. The vegetable garden, as it could be watered all the year round, produced tomatoes and leafy green vegetables (lettuce, ordinary spinach and the succulent climbing spinach) and above all pumpkins (Cucurbita pepo) which are fast-growing, coarse ground-trailing plants providing 'squash', the yellow pulp from which are made 'pumpkin pies'. Ours were so fast-growing that they threatened to attack the bungalow's rear

BACK TO KADUNA

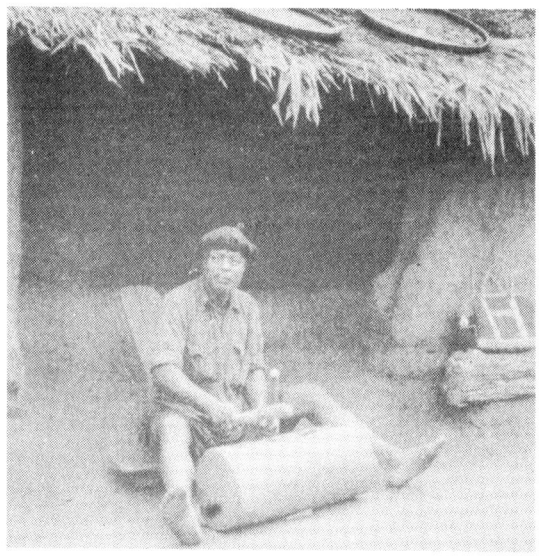

Drum when beaten summons workers in the fields.

balcony at a rate of about two-and-a-half feet per day. The biggest pumpkin we grew weighed 56 lbs., a lot of 'pie'! On that rear balcony Mary had her herbs growing in pots (basil, chives, rosemary, fennel and others).

Bawa had about one-quarter acre of the compound on which he could grow what he wanted. Over the years he rotated crops of groundnuts with cassava and sweet potatoes.

For shade we planted a number of flame tree seedlings which grew so fast that within three years Diana derived great fun from climbing them. The Deputy Director of WAITR, Tam Nash, kindly gave us a cutting of 'golden shower' which soon covered our front verandah with a mat of delightful orange-yellow blooms. Mary's pride and joy were hollyhocks which she coaxed to grow remarkably well along the front wing of the bungalow outside our bedroom.

Fruit Trees in Bornu Province

On my return to Maiduguri after my first visit to Lake Chad I had called on the senior NA agricultural assistant for Bornu

Province, Mallam Lawan. He was very well educated and professionally extremely proficient. I explained that I was sure the Kanuri and Shuwa Arabs of the region, and probably the townsfolk of Maiduguri were suffering from illnesses caused by deficiencies of vitamins A and C. He knew what I was talking about. I asked if it would be possible to get the rural families to plant a citrus tree in each compound, or guavas and mangoes (Mangifira indira) which were known to the Bornu peoples but seldom grown. Mallam Lawan said it would be possible to grow these fruits quite easily using composted night-soil as fertiliser (cattle dung was used as kitchen fuel in this area or for facing the walls of the domestic mud huts) provided the people would water the seedlings until they were well established, a habit he had not yet succeeded in persuading them was worth while. But he could try again using his own extension staff to start the cultivation in certain selected village headmen's compounds. He would need help in establishing a citrus and mango nursery at his own headquarters on the road to Lake Chad just north of Maiduguri. With the help of Phil Chambers this nursery was built up with contributions from Shendam.

The next question to answer was whether to give the seedlings free to the village headman, my own view, or to charge a small amount such as 3d (threepence) a seedling which Mallam considered would make the people believe there was some worth attached to the venture. After four years the fruit trees had been so successfully established that all compound heads, not only village headmen, were willing to buy seedlings from the nursery for 2/6d (two shillings and sixpence) each, such was the profit made by their wives selling the fruit in the Maiduguri area and other major markets.

Replacing Roots by Rice
We had tried to repeat the fruit-growing activities so successful in Bornu in and around Sokoto, unfortunately with much less success. For some years the Sokoto NA agricultural and forestry activities had been directed towards the afforestation of the headwaters of the streams in the area of Argungu, Qwandu, Bernin Kebbi and Gwotoma, which ran into the Sokoto River to prevent erosion; the building up of check dams and teaching of contour farming and irrigation, and the planting of rice grown as

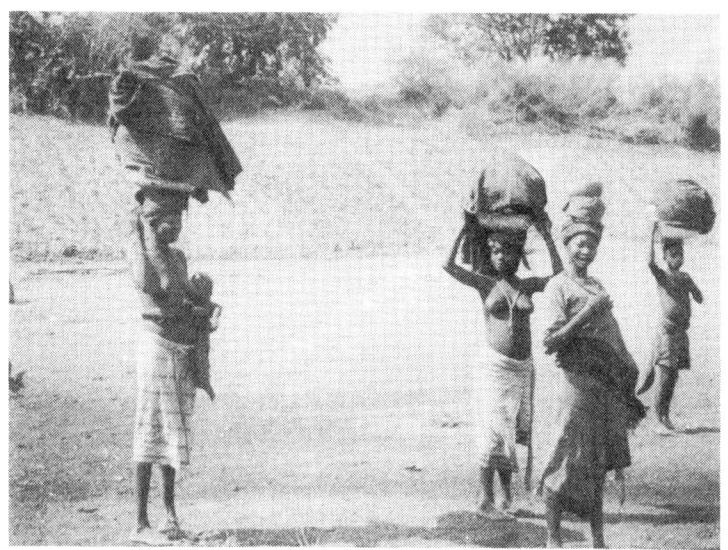

En route to market, five miles north of Yelwa.

an upland crop on alluvial soil left at the end of the wet season. An agriculture officer had had the bright idea that mechanised ploughing, rather than having this alluvial 'fadama', would help the farmers with growing rice. This was even less successful, and more liable to produce erosion, than the experiment in mechanical ploughing to increase the amount of guinea corn grown on flat non-alluvial land at Mokwa in Niger Province. Rice was not necessary to improve the energy and protein intakes of the Sokoto Fulani who, except in times of drought, ate well on the traditional diet of upland finger millet, bulrush millet and guinea corn. Some rice was eaten in the area but it was grown mainly as a cash crop.

When I had first gone to Bida I had found that the cultivation of deep water rice was starting at Badeggi. This production expanded rapidly but was used as a cash crop for sale to the trading firms rather than as a food crop. As milling facilities were not available, the rice was home produced, pounded and parboiled before consumption or selling to markets south of Niger Province where it was needed to replace root crops.

The message that rice production should be increased south of the Niger-Benue line still needed to be emphasised and, following a tentative start, planning was needed to implement the simple maxim — 'more fruit and vegetables north of the line of the rivers, replace roots by rice south of that line'.

The Regional Nutrition Committees

All three regions nominally had nutrition committees established away back in the 1920s and 1930s on the initiative of Dr W. E. McCulloch in the Northern Provinces and by Dr D. G. Fitzgerald Moore in the Southern Provinces. All were moribund when the FNU was formed in 1953. Their original function had been to advise the DMS in Lagos of the prevalence of diseases which, at the time of these committees' formation, were well known to be caused by deficiencies of specific nutrients, e.g. goitre, rickets, scurvy and beri-beri. McCulloch is quite specific in his detailed article (Government Printer, Lagos, 1930) on the'Dietaries of the Hausas and of the Town Fulani' that he had not seen a case of pellegra in Nigeria, and that in the general population vitamin B deficiency was not prevalent. Beri-beri was seldom seen although 'epidemics' of this disease had occurred in prisons when the staple foodstuffs had been changed from millet and guinea corn to 'polished' rice. Sore tongues, cracks at the margins of the lips and irritative inflammation of the external genitalia had not yet been attributed to vitamin B (riboflavin) deficiency.

Our surveys in Niger and Delta Provinces and in the other seven areas in different ecological zones had clarified the clinical situation in relationship to food consumption, energy, protein and other nutrient requirements. They had also shown that the Medical Department, acting on its own, could not do much more than treat cases of nutritional deficiency diseases in an empirical fashion in dispensaries or in hospitals. What was needed to improve the nutritional situation in the country was close co-operation between federal and regional government administrations, in particular their treasuries, and the departments of agriculture, forestry, fisheries and education and the information services. In this overall picture the greatest help the departments of medicine could give was through a great improvement and concentration on preventive public health measures to reduce infections and parasitism.

The Federal Government had demonstrated positive interest in ascertaining the state of food supplies in relation to health budgeting for the formation of the Federal Nutrition Unit and in the concept of inter-departmental co-operation towards increasing and improving the production and distribution of staple foodstuffs. The regional governments, particularly in the north and east, established what we now call Food Production and Nutrition Committees. In the Western Region, although a Food Production and Nutrition Committee was formed, co-operation between the concerned departments tended to be over-written by the Department of Medicine of Ibadan University, where many of the staff, expatriates and Nigerian alike, however competent clinicians or biochemists they were, could not see the necessity of going beyond the stage of hospital therapy to prevent the development of under-nutrition and malnutrition. The wards were always full of such patients drawn from the shanty towns surrounding Ibadan and I eventually reached the conclusion that both biochemists and clinicians alike used these patients, quite unnecessarily, more or less as guinea-pigs whereby to establish their own reputations in laboratories and wards. Such an approach was anathema to me, as were certain of the individuals concerned.

An important factor which was found to affect the diets consumed in the different parts of Nigeria and hence their nutritional value was the inter-regional movement of major food crops. Such phenomena as the transport of sun-dried and smoked fish from Lake Chad to the markets in the overcrowded towns of the Eastern Region, or the apparent fact that a greater quantity of cowpeas than that produced in the Eastern and Western Regions was consumed in those regions, were conclusions drawn from the FNU surveys and considered by the Northern Region Food Production and Nutrition Committee.

It is encouraging to find that surveys of food consumption in relation to nutritional status and prevalence of energy protein are still being carried out by the Nigerian staff of the more newly formed universities. Their results do not show much improvement in the general state of affairs and, I think, indicate a loss of the inter-ministerial co-operation described which took place in 1959. Without this co-operation between food-producing ministries, education authorities and public health activities of ministries of health, the eradication of under and malnutrition, infectious diseases and parasitism will not be achieved.

Increasing Contacts with International Affairs and Agencies
The supposition that lack of dietary protein of good quality was the prime cause of the syndrome variously known as kwashiorkor, marasmus, marasinic kwashiorkor, starch food dystrophy, protein malnutrition — call it what you will — was growing apace. This concept was believed not only by physicians, paediatricians, white-faced tropical medicine men, biochemists and pathologists who worked in developing countries but also by the same categories of people who had never worked in the tropics who used various experimental animals for their feeding trials, using diets deficient in protein but adequate in energy (calories).

Protein-rich Foods
Food technologists and manufacturers of infant foods such as Glaxo became interested in the subject. UNICEF began to distribute any dried skimmed milk (DSM) it could acquire from governmental surpluses donated to the fund as part of their assessed contributions to the UN Organisation. Such distributions covered the free issue of DSM to mothers and pre-school children and school and hospital feeding programmes in many developing countries, of which Nigeria was not one. The intention was admirable provided (a) the hypothesis that protein deficiency was the cause of 'kwashiorkor' and (b) that the DSM reached the target group and was not diverted to those who did not need it such as the families of local administrators, fathers and older healthy children. Therefore close supervision of these distribution programmes was frequently required but was not always provided. The Nigerian FNU could only give advice to dispensaries, schools and hospitals; it could not act in a supervisory capacity so I advised against accepting DSM.

The provision of protein concentrates was being developed in several countries using as a base suitable foodstuffs readily available in the needy countries themselves. This approach seemed sensible to me and the Federal Government of Nigeria, through the representative of UNICEF, became interested in producing some such product and asked the Federal Nutrition Unit for ideas on the subject. In about 1950 a dairy to make butter from cow's milk had been set up in Vom in the Plateau Province near Jos. Some time in 1953 or 1954 I had noted that the buttermilk from the dairy was being channelled away from the building in an open concrete drain. The local Old World Vultures (Accipitridae) were drinking this effluent with some relish and made me think such waste might be put to good use. Samples analysed in the FNU showed that the buttermilk had a proximate composition of protein (N x 6.35) 20 per cent fat 0.5 per cent and carbohydrate 70 per cent or .365 kcal/100 g, with plentiful calcium, iron, thiamine, nicotinic acid and riboflavin (Government Chemist, London).

On the basis of this information UNICEF agreed with a request from the Northern Regional Government to put up a roller-drying milk plant at Vom in an attempt to dry the wasted buttermilk. The plant was ready to work in 1956 and a Dutchman, expert in roller-drying whole or skimmed milk, Mr Hoelgaard, who had erected the plant near the Vom dairy, started trials roller-drying buttermilk which he had not done before. One difficulty was to collect a sufficient amount of the buttermilk to run over the rollers for some time while he changed the temperatures up and down and altered the speed of rotation. So he eventually built a large storage tank, specially cooled to store up to 200 litres of buttermlk. This was an unexpected extra expense on the UNICEF allocation. Any supplement to the original vote had to be authorised by the next UNICEF Executive Board meeting months away. All this administrative palaver took time and I began to feel the frustration suffered by so many personnel working in international organisations.

Meantime, on Nigeria's own initiative, we started to make a high quality groundnut flour (GNF) at Zaria. Groundnuts were in plentiful supply and an enterprising Lebanese called Kahlil had started to produce a groundnut press cake as a by-product to the lucrative production of groundnut oil. (For groundnut in American read peanut!) This cake was primarily for use in animal feeding, mainly of pigs! It was an extraordinary fact that pigs (American hogs!) were reared in large numbers in Kano, the Moslem heart of Northern Nigeria, where the climate suits them. It was economically more rewarding to breed and rear them in the north, slaughter them and rail the carcasses to the south in refrigerated vans. I asked Khalil to try to refine his groundnut press cake to make a product which was cleaner and more finely ground so that it might be used for human consumption. He tried, but without any financial stimulus, which I could not offer him, he went on with his groundnut cake for 'feed' as opposed to food.

It so happened that our friend Ronald Berriff had been posted from Lagos to Kaduna as the first Permanent Under Secretary to the Northern Regional Ministry of Trade and Industry, just converted from a department. He found that his predecessor, as Director of the Department of Trade and Industry, had organised a unit in Zaria, fifty miles from Kaduna, where shea butter was being produced for sale to the trading companies, mainly UAC, for export. As this food product was not an important item of diet the FNU had no objection to its sale overseas. Berriff found that certain equipment for the production of finely milled flour had been ordered, possibly from the Northern Region Development Corporation (NRDC) for use, maybe, in grinding sorghum and millet. The NRDC worked closely with the Marketing Boards whose function was to cushion the farmers against unpredictable fluctuations in world prices of their exported products, such as groundnuts, cocoa, palm produce and so on. The Marketing Boards from accumulated reserves, also sponsored development projects such as irrigation schemes, supply of fertilisers and equipment for technical development through the regional development corporations.

Ron Berriff and I had close consultations, together and with others concerned, about the use of the flour mill which was lying idle in charge of the Ministry of Trade and Industry. I wanted it to be used to process groundnut press cake into a finely ground product suitable for human consumption. Eventually it was agreed that whole groundnuts would be purchased from the Marketing Boards and that the various plants at Zaria would express the oil and resell it for export overseas, while the press cake would be processed by the new mill. This was agreed and soon an excellent quality of flour was being produced under the supervision of a first-class technical engineer recruited by the Ministry, Mr Jack Brown, a specialist in food processing.

The roller drying of the buttermilk was not going too well at the UNICEF plant at Vom on account of shortage of supplies from the dairy. A decision had to be made about collecting whole milk from the cattle herdsmen on the plateau within reach of the Vom roller-drying plant. There was a rumour around that the wives of so many of the herdsmen made butter for their own use and threw away the buttermilk. Would it not be a good idea to try to buy this milk, after the calves had been weaned, allow the dairy to separate it producing skimmed milk and then roller dry the skimmed milk together with the GNF to produce a product I wanted to christen ARLAC (AR from *arachis*, groundnut; LAC for *lactis*, Latin for milk)?

Berriff was cautious about this approach and wanted some expert opinion from overseas. Mr Robert Cooper, then the UNICEF milk expert based in the Paris office (which was also responsible for the African region of UNICEF), was asked if he could attend a meeting, first in Kaduna and then at Vom, to discuss the matter with a representative of the Food and Agriculture Organisation of the UN Animal Protection and Health Division, Mr Neil Reid and Mr Geof Wilson, Northern Region Veterinary Department. News spreads fast and it so happened the Dr W. F. J. Cuthbertson of Glaxo Research Ltd., UK, also arrived to attend the meeting. If meeting it could be called! It took place on the lawn in front of our verandah at 14 Cunliffe Close on 7 April 1953 at drinks time. Mary was at home for our children's Easter holidays. I had found accommodation for all the visitors in the Kaduna Catering Rest House, and for the next week at Hill Station, Jos, whence they could try to assess the milk supply situation on the Plateau.

It had been agreed at the Cunliffe Close meeting that the production of roller-dried skimmed milk should be undertaken if the available supplies of whole milk were likely within fifty miles of Vom and that transport should be sent out from the dairy to prearranged collecting points. After a few days the team agreed that sufficient milk would be available at a price per gallon which was satisfactory to the herdsmen. The dairy was not happy that it should be converted to a creamery but political factors prevailed. An effort was made to roller dry a mixture of three parts to one part of GNF to DSM. This was a failure and eventually the CNF from Zaria was sent by road to Vom to be mixed directly with the DSM in the above proportions, the dry mixer being called ARLAC. In May 1958 the chairman of Glaxo, Sir Harry Jephcott, and his wife, paid a visit to Kano with Dr Cuthbertson where Mary and I met them. We found out then that Glaxo was about to market a product based on ground nut flour and milk and called ARAMA. When I asked Cuth, as he was always known, why ARAMA had been chosen as a name, he replied, 'Because the word is not very rude in any of the West African dialects.'

From its inception ARLAC was to be used in government organisations, such as health department dispensaries, hospitals, maternal and child health clinics, school feeding programmes and the mission stations for a nominal sum. It had never been intended for general sale until the volume of production had saturated the above objectives. Now, maybe, the future ARAMA would be a competitor. ARLAC was an economic product. The cost of GNF at Zaria was (at current prices and in US cents for UNICEF's easy interpretation) 6-7 cents per lb, the DSM at Vom 28 cents per lb, ARLAC 12 cents per lb at Vom, compared to 56 cents per lb for imported dried milk.

Thus Nigeria had produced a protein rich food to supplement starchy diets, hopefully to prevent the now fashionable 'protein malnutrition' and possibly to act as a curative agent.

Possibility of Work outside Nigeria

In April 1958 Dr R. C. (Jim) Burgess, Chief of the Nutrition Section of WHO HQ in Geneva, had written to me asking me to put my name forward to WHO for an appointment in his section. This I had done.

He wrote to Nigeria asking Mary and me to visit Geneva the next time we were going on leave. This we did in July 1958, staying for the first of innumerable times at the Cornavin Hotel in Geneva. Jim saw me in his office at the Palais des Nations, the building which was supposed to become the first HQ of the League of Nations. He explained that, at the moment, the number of British people employed by WHO was greatly in excess of the UK quota so he could not offer me a job immediately but he would have my application reviewed by the WHO administration from time to time and possibly it would be accepted sometime in the future. How long could I wait? I said I did not know but that independence of Nigeria was on the cards within the next few years and no one knew what would happen to expatriates thereafter. I never got that appointment which was ultimately filled by Edouard de Mayer from IRSAC in the Belgian Congo.

BACK TO KADUNA

At the Lwiru seminar in 1959 Dr J. M. Latsky, Chief Adviser on Nutrition to the Ministry of Health, Pretoria, Union of South Africa, asked me if I would like to join the South African Nutrition Research Unit of the Ministry of Health in Pretoria. I did not have any difficulty in saying no to this kind offer. Latsky was African, was a charming man but I had not any urge to learn his language.

On the airplane between Usumbura (now Busumbura) and Leopoldville (now Kinshasa) I was seated next to Marcel Autret of FAO. He thanked me for my contribution to the seminar at Lwiru and wondered if I would be interested in becoming a staff member of the Nutrition Division of the Food and Agriculture Organisation of the United Nations. I told him that I had already been asked by Jim Burgess to join WHO and that this was still on the cards. Had FAO got too big a British element on its staff quota? He said that if it had he and Aykroyd could get around it. This did not sound like Aykroyd to me, so the question was left in abeyance.

When I reached Kaduna from the Congo at the beginning of December 1959 I was told that a certain Dr Lewthwaite from UK had visited WAITR, Kaduna, was now touring Nigeria and would return to Nigeria early in the New Year 1960. Platt had told me about Lewthwaite, who was one of the medical advisers to the Colonial Office, and was a member of the Medical Research Council of the Privy Council (MRC). When finally we met in, I think, January 1960, he told me that he knew my uncle Landsborough Thomson very well (not surprising as Uncle Lance had been secretary to the MRC since its inception in 1919) and that they both would like me to take over the directorship of the East African Medical Survey and Research Unit at Mwanza, Tanganyika, on the banks of Lake Victoria, which was supported by MRC funds. Dr Eric Holmes had been trying to introduce nutrition research into the unit's programme, which had previously been concentrating on studies of filariasis. I had seen enough of filariasis in the Delta Province of Western Nigeria to decide at once that it would probably be better to think in terms of the international organisations rather than a swamp on the southern bank of Lake Victoria, Tanganyika. So I told Dr Lewthwaite that I was already committed to FAO or WHO, whichever came up first with a post for me. Dr Lewthwaite was not too happy about this answer, but my mind was made up against the Mwanza appointment. This decision was voluntary and not dictated by the whims of Chance!

*The WHO Protein Advisory Group and the
US Committee on Protein Malnutrtion*
The emphasis on the importance of protein-rich food supplements, made from indigenous foodstuffs, locally processed, for the consumption of infants, their mothers and toddlers very naturally gave WHO, and in particular its Nutrition Section, some worries about the value and safety of using such products in maternal and child health feeding around the world. Paediatricians and physicians concerned by the reports of childhood malnutrition in developing countries were also interested in the formation of an organisation of some sort to check on the safety of using locally grown and formulated protein foods.

As a result of this interest in the subject, and following discussions between Dr Charles Glen King, W. J. Darby and Paul Gyorgy with Dr M. G. Candau, Director-General of WHO, and Dr R. C. (Jim) Burgess, Chief of Nutrition Section of WHO, the WHO Protein Advisory Group (PAG) was established in 1955. Its object was to advise WHO on the identification, study and development of protein-rich foods 'which are being or can be produced or made available for human feeding in areas now protein deficient. Such foods must be economically feasible, preferably locally available, readily acceptable, nutritious, free of toxic products or substances, nutritionally useful . . . and possess good storage qualities under rather simple conditions' (quote from the first PAG Bulletin, dated 1 January 1956). The PAG's first members were Dr William J. Darby, Co-ordinator, Director, Division of Nutrition, Vanderbilt University, Nashville, Tennessee; Dr L. Emmett Holt, Jnr., Professor of Paediatrics, New York University School of Medicine, New York; Dr Benjamin Platt, Human Nutrition Research Unit, National Institute for Medical Research, London; Dr Paul Gyorgy, Professor of Paediatrics, University of Pennsylvania, Philadelphia; and Dr Eric K. Cruikshank (son of my Professor of Bacteriology at Aberdeen), Professor of Medicine, University College of the West Indies, Jamaica.

It was not until 1960 that FAO and UNICEF also became sponsors of the PAG.

Of much great importance to the Nigerian Food and Nutrition Unit was the early recognition that a great deal of research on potentially suitable foodstuffs would be needed around the world. To meet this need the Food and Nutrition Board of the US National Academy of Sciences/National Research Council appointed a Committee on Protein Malnutrition with Dr Henry Sebrell of Columbia University, New York, as chairman, the members being Dr Grace Goldsmith of Tulane University; Dr Paul Gyorgy; Mr G. E. Hilbert of the US Department of Agriculture; Dr J. M. Hundley, National Institutes of Health, Betheseda, Maryland, and Dr W. J. Darby. This committee was supported by a grant of $550,000 from the Rockefeller Foundation and an allocation of $300,000 from the Executive Board of UNICEF. The money was to be used for laboratory and clinical testing, process development, safety and acceptability trials of protein-rich foods. After a visit to Nigeria by Drs Bill Darby, Jim Hundley, Mark Hegsted and Martha Trulson (nutritionist with Dr Stare at the Harvard School of Public Health) in January 1957, it was decided to grant the Nigerian FNU an initial sum of US $17,000 to determine the net protein utilisation of two protein-rich foods prepared in the United States, namely groundnut flour (GNF) and dried skimmed milk (DSM), their efficacy and safety as supplements to the diets of schoolchildren and their value in the treatment of infants and toddlers suffering from protein malnutrition (as it was then called). I asked for, and was granted, permission to use ARLAC, produced in Nigeria, in the treatment of protein malnutrition, in infants and young children.

This financial windfall was repeated in 1958 when the FNU was granted an additional US $20,000 after Professor Ben Platt had visited the Unit in Kaduna, and spent a very pleasant week living with us in our bungalow while inspecting the laboratory facilities and work. I had met him in Kano and driven him by road to Kaduna and he insisted on stopping at all the markets in the villages or at the roadside. He wanted to get a feeling of what foodstuffs were available in the Sudan and Guinea savannah zones through which we passed en route.

Introducing ARLAC into the Community
We had established a Nutrition Unit Clinic in a native compound in Tudan Wada, a small hamlet three miles south of Kaduna where

a Mother and Child Health Centre (MCHC) had been opened by the Native Authority some years before. The mothers and the children who attended it were mostly of the Gwari tribe, who preferred to be examined in an environment more like their own homes than be bothered by the formalities of the Kaduna General Hospital. Any infants and children considered by the staff to be suffering from malnutrition of any form were referred to the FNU Clinic. If I considered the infants or toddlers were acutely ill they were transferred to the General Hospital where the DMS had kindly allocated me a small ward for the study and treatment of such acute cases until they could be returned to the Tudan Wada clinic and the care of European nursing sisters and NA Community Services Nurses. These dedicated nursing sisters, who worked at Tudan Wada and supervised the diets at the compound where we did N balance studies on men, were wives of administrative officers or other colonial civil servants stationed in Kaduna who had volunteered for this work. All of them were well qualified and experienced in UK in general nursing (SRN), some in obstetrics and gynaecology or in dietetrics, making them excellent assistants in our work. They were paid a small salary from the Rockefeller Foundation grant but would have carried out these duties without payment merely for something worthwhile to do. Their husbands did not go on tour in the bush often, if at all, and their wives all enjoyed learning something of the basic facts of tribal life in Nigeria, something many of their office-bound husbands never learnt.

The mothers of the infants and children suffering from moderate or mild forms of protein malnutrition (kwashiorkor, marasmus) reported to the Nutrition Clinic in Tudan Wada weekly so that their children could be weighed, physically checked, and given a 2 lb. packet of ARLAC when necessary. The ARLAC was fed at a level of 6g protein/kg as a supplement to their home diets. Intercurrent infections were treated at home or as in-patients in the Nutrition Unit Clinic in the Tudan Wada compound. This procedure was much preferable to the mothers than the palaver of admission to Kaduna General Hospital. A nursing sister and a Nigerian nurse visited the children's homes to ensure that the dietary supplement was being given correctly to them by their mothers. The results of this supplementary feeding programme showed that the babies who continued to take ARLAC from the age of nine months to two years lost a little weight for the first two months due to the disappearance of oedema. From eleven to twenty-four months they gained weight rapidly and by then had overtaken, in weight, infants of the same age who had never suffered from protein malnutrition.

Farewell to Nigeria

The work on man's protein requirements carried out by the FNU was the end of my medical research work as far as I was concerned. I had decided to leave Nigeria before the country was granted full independence from the United Kingdom and the Chief Medical Adviser to the Federal Government, Sir Samuel Manuwa, and the Governor-General, Sir James Robertson, had agreed to my retirement after Northern Nigeria had received its own regional independence. Sir Bryan Sharwood-Smith had retired in September 1957 and been succeeded as Governor by Sir Gawain Bell, who earlier had served in the Sudan. On 15 March 1959 he had appointed me, a Federal Nigerian civil servant, to be a member of the Public Service Commission (PSC) of the Northern Region, under the chairmanship of Dennis Hibbert, lately Deputy Director of Education, Northern Nigeria. The members included the ex-Minister Alhaji Bello, Kano, and the editor of the newspaper *Gaskiya Ta Fi Kwabo* (The Truth costs but a Penny), Alhaji Abubakar Imam. He was later chairman of the PSC.

The PSC had numerous functions but, as its members were carefully chosen for their competence, honesty and impartiality, its primary but unwritten function was to control nepotism when civil service appointments had to be made, and to select the most suitable candidates for such appointments from those put forward by the various ministries and departments. Another important and time-consuming task given to the PSC was the election of students to take up scholarships granted by the government, or financed from other public sources, at overseas universities or colleges, mostly at that time in UK.

In addition to the work of the FNU, writing up the papers mentioned above, and the small amount of 'general practice' I still carried on looking after friends and their families and the staff at Government House, I did not have much spare time. However, both Mary and I, now that both children were at boarding schools in UK, missed the touring in the 'bush' which had taken up so much of our time for so many years. It was suggested by Ronald Berriff to Mary that she apply for the job of confidential secretary to Bob Mortimore, the general manager of the rapidly expanding Kaduna Textiles factory, an appointment she fulfilled very well for the last two and a half years we lived in Kaduna. She still states with satisfaction that she paid for Diana's school fees during that time — a great help to our family finances and very mentally rewarding for Mary, giving her a good excuse to avoid the coffee-party, bridge-playing set of wives, while allowing time for tennis at the club in the early evenings. She became a regular partner of the Attorney-General, Hedley Marshall, and together they did well in the various competitions. I started playing cricket again, the first time since before the war, and I was not entirely unsuccessful.

In January 1960 Sir Samuel had sent me a Nigerian civil service medical officer, a Yoruba called Oshodi, who was reputed to be interested in nutrition having worked on the subject in the laboratories and wards of Ibadan General Hospital. He was to take over the FNU from me when I left the country. I soon found out he had not had any experience in the 'bush'. We still had a little of the Rockefeller grant money left so, when I finally left Nigeria for the last time in August 1960, I left Peter Phillips in charge of the grant with instructions to do a final feeding trial to determine the effect on NPU of the so-called 'imbalance' of leucine and iso-leucine in guinea corn (sorghum). Peter himself had not made up his mind whether to stay on in Kaduna or retire to UK. In the end he kept the FNU going for about one year after I left. Dr Oshodi was then left without a biochemist, without any plans for follow-up survey work which would have been useful. Nor was he interested in stimulating the Regional Nutrition Committees to continue their co-ordination of food production in relation to food consumption and clinical status. In the end the FNU was withdrawn from Kaduna and its excellent accommodation in WAITR to Lagos where it was purged of many of its staff and located in a small wing of Medical Headquarters on the Marina, Lagos.

I had suggested and made arrangements for a food consumption and clinical survey of a sample of the lower-income groups in Lagos. Dr Oshodi liked the idea as he could return to the town and he did try his best to carry out what was a very difficult

BACK TO KADUNA

job. But in the end I do not believe this Lagos survey was ever completed.

While I had been Federal Adviser on Nutrition to the Nigerian Government I had frequently visited both the Nutrition Division of FAO in Rome and the Nutrition Section of WHO at the organisation's HQ in Geneva. In keeping with the old plan followed by CCTA and my first DMS in Lagos (Jerry Walker) to keep the international agencies out of Nigeria, FAO and WHO had agreed not to visit Nigeria unless I requested assistance. WHO never did send a nutrition representative to Nigeria while I was there, but for FAO Marcel Autret had paid a short visit to Kano, where we looked at Khalil's groundnut oil and meal plant. As he had arrived in the country unasked, I thought he should see what we had to offer in the way of food and nutrition activities. He said he could not visit either Zaria or Vom to see the preparation of ARLAC nor could he visit our laboratories and clinics at WAITR or in Tudan Wada. He went on to Lagos from Kano, I believe en route to the Congo, but I never knew his final destination. Later he told me he had had a suit of clothes removed from his luggage while staying in the Lagos airport 'hotel' at Ikeja about which he was very angry. Later we were visited in Kaduna by a member of the FAO Nutrition staff in Rome, Marcel Ganzin. He stayed with us in our bungalow for a few days and seemed interested, up to a point, in our work on man's protein requirements, although he was obviously not up to date with the subject. He had once been in the French Colonial Medical Service as a 'pharmacien' at the Pasteur Institute in Brazzaville, French Equatorial Africa. Autret also had been a 'pharmacien' in French Indo-China in the Far East, based on Saigon. He and his wife had been prisoners of war of the Japanese and this misfortune had prevented him doing any practical work during that period. Thus at the end of the war in the Far East he was quite out of date with the important nutritional studies which had been carried out in Europe and North America.

When it became known to WHO and FAO that I was about to retire from the Colonial Medical Service, WHO still did not have a vacancy for me because its UK staff quota was oversubscribed. However, Dr Aykroyd, who was about to retire from FAO, was able to put my name forward to the Director-General, Dr B. R.

Sen. By May 1960 it had been agreed that I would be appointed to the Nutrition Division of FAO towards the end of that year.

This fact appeared to stimulate FAO's interest in the development of FAO/UNICEF supported programmes in Nigeria. Early in July 1960 I was asked to meet a certain temporary staff member of the FAO Nutrition Divisions, a Mexican by the name of Joachim Cravioto, at Kano Airport, and to study with him the possibility of starting 'applied nutrition projects' in different areas of the country. He did not appear to know anything about the very similar programme that had been developed in the Kontagora and Bida areas in 1947-49 and which we had abandoned as a wrong approach to solving the problems of under-nutrition and malnutrition for want of local, provincial, regional and central government support. Nor had he or the Nutrition Division heard of the 1959 Economic Survey of Nigeria which contained so much information about the development of agriculture and fisheries in relation to the nutrition of the peoples of Nigeria. He had not read any of my earlier papers published in the British Journal of Nutrition between 1948 and 1959. This was not his fault because neither had most of the staff of the Nutrition Division of FAO read them. His visit and approach on behalf of the nutrition Division made me wonder if I had made a wise decision to join FAO. WHO would have been a much more suitable organisation for me to work in despite my conviction of the importance of agricultural development in different ecological zones in meeting the nutritional needs of the populations of developing countries. However, chance had again played its part and I was destined for FAO.

Dr Carvioto was still with us when Mary and I visited Lagos earlier in July 1960 to bid farewell to our colleagues and friends there. Mary had been asked to find herself a present to be given to her by Kaduna Textiles staff and selected a shortwave portable wireless set which worked very well, even in USA.

Towards the end of July Mary flew home to England for the children's summer holidays after we had been presented by the Federal Nutrition Unit staff with some exceedingly well-made ebony figures, some of the best examples of this form of Nigerian art I have ever seen. In 14 Cunliffe Close our houseboys, myself and the PWD packed and crated our belongings which had accumulated in Nigeria since 1946/47. They were destined to be sent by sea and collected and stored in London by Cox's and King's until such time as we knew where to put them.

Mary, Christopher and Diana stayed in a small private hotel, 'Winterdene', near Mary's father's house, a comfortable place we had used from time to time while in Bournemouth on leave from Nigeria.

After several farewell parties in Kaduna, including a very cheerful lunch at Government House with Sir Gawain and Lady Bell, I flew back to join the family at Winterdene in the middle of August 1960.

CHAPTER 10

Developing Personal Roots in England

As I had decided to retire from Nigeria and would not join FAO until the end of 1960, Mary and I thought the period between September and December 1960 should be spent looking for a house which the family could call 'home'. Since our wedding in October 1940 we had moved from one rented house to another during the Battle of Britain and my service in Combined Operations and with the Guards Armoured Division until the end of the war and my final demobilisation. Often we had stayed with kind relatives while on leave or in boarding houses or small hotels like Winterdene. We had pleasant memories of living in Nigerian government accommodation in Bida, Warri, Lagos and particularly in 14 Cunliffe Close, Kaduna. Mary's step-sister, 'Dick' Prothero, had been particularly kind to Mary and the children while I was overseas in the army, as had her Aunt Vera Eaton.

With the aid of a co-operative house agency firm we were very lucky in finding a small house in Dorset, about 500 yards from the Ferndown Golf Club, by the beginning of October. It is called 'Trackway', or some still call it 'The Trackway', as it had a deep ditch which still runs across the seventeenth fairway and then divided, on the rough track outside our gate, into a ditch then ran on towards Verwood to the north and the third branch went towards Ringwood to the east. These ditches are reputed to have been used by the brandy smuggler, Gulliver, on his way inland from the coast near Poole where he met the small French boats at night, at Lilliput. A nearby house is called 'Gullivers'.

I was lucky to be able to buy the house by commuting a part of my Nigerian pension for £5,000. With carpets, curtains, and some furniture the owner did not want to take away, I paid £7,000 for the lot in 1960. We still live in Trackway which Mary and I hold in trust for Christopher and Diana. When we bought it

DEVELOPING PERSONAL ROOTS IN ENGLAND

Christopher was nearly nineteen and Diana was twelve-and-a-half years old.

The reason we chose Ferndown in Dorset to buy a house was that Scotland we considered would be too cold a place and Mary would be close to her father, then in his eighty-eighth year. Also we had other friends and relations in Dorset. 'Trackway' is a small house with only a sitting room, dining room, and small kitchen, two double bedrooms and one small single bedroom. Yet it suits D. and C. when they come to see us, very well and we cannot put up more than two separate visitors or one married couple and a single person.

We had the packing cases sent down from London and started to settle in. Some of our wedding presents, for some reason now forgotten, had been stored in 81 High Street, Old Aberdeen, since 1940. Twenty years on we were able to have them sent down to Trackway in some of those nice old-fashioned tea boxes. By the end of November we were reasonably well settled into our first and, so far, only home of our own.

During this period of settling into Trackway, and before I became a staff member of FAO, Marcel Autret, the Director, asked me if I could act as a consultant on the food and nutrition aspects of agricultural development in Northern Nigeria. Apparently the regional government had requested the UN Special Fund to send an international team to examine the situation current in 1960 and to make recommendations for future action, with the hope of getting grants to fund particular development projection the overall agricultural field. This team was co-ordinated by FAO, Rome. My participation in the project for three weeks was to help the team write its up to the final report. As I had been working along the lines of the team's terms of reference for more than twelve years it was thought I might be of some help. Thus I spent three weeks in October/November 1960 in Kaduna, where the team was based, living in the Catering Rest House. I had left Kaduna only two months before, and it was too soon to send me back, as I was received with very lavish hospitality offered by my old friends, from the Governor, Sir Gawain Bell, downwards, and this was a severe tax on my staying power. However, I was able to give the UNSDP team some up-to-date information on the food and nutrition aspects of the region, the type of projects they should recommend for support and refer it to government proposals which

I knew were already awaiting funding. This was the approach the financial secretary was expecting from me.

It was obvious that the team, which had only been allowed to spend about three months in Nigeria, had not gathered a true background to the food and nutrition situation, thus I believe I was able to help in formulating certain proposals acceptable to the team's leader and to the country. Naturally they were along the lines I had already proposed to the government — more fruit and vegetables in the arid northern areas and replace roots (yams and cassava) by rice in the southern part of the region and country, and to increase the availability for consumption of fresh or cured meat and fish throughout all ecological zones. The altered patterns of basic food production should be accompanied by better control of food distribution and a reduction of waste by improved storage facilities.

I saw that the Federal Nutrition Unit was still working quite well in WAITR and had discussions with Peter Phillips. Dr Oshodi was working in Lagos on the food consumption and health survey I had started only a few months ago.

At the end of the three weeks I travelled to Rome with the team where the report was presented to the Assistant Director General of the Agricultural Department and to the interested staff members of the various Divisions in that department, e.g. Animal Production and Health, Land and Water, Fisheries, Forestry, Nutrition and others. It was reasonably well received and some of the projects recommended were eventually funded by the UNSPD.

After continuing the settling-in process at Trackway and seeing friends who lived locally, mainly the Handbys and Andersons who we had first met in Warri in 1949/50 we spent Christmas and the New Year in our own home *en famille*. I started playing golf on the Ferndown course but not for long. On 19 January 1961 I flew from London to Rome to join the Nutrition Division of FAO.

Mary's father died on 27 January 1961. He had been ill for only a few weeks and Mary brought her step-mother, Mabel, back from the funeral to stay a few days in Trackway, where she was our first visitor. I did not go back to Bournemouth for the funeral as Mary and Mabel did not think this was necessary and might upset the process of settling into FAO.

I went to Rome in the winter of 1961 and Mary joined me in a pensione near the Piazza Barberini. We started to get to know

Rome by walking around at the weekends and having dinner occasionally in small restaurants around the Piazza Barberini area.

I soon got to know the staff of the Nutrition Division. Dr Wallace Aykroyd, its Director since the inception of FAO in October 1945, its spell in Washington until 1951 and since its move to Rome that year, had retired at the age of sixty, a few months before I arrived in Rome, and, after considerable discussion, the Frenchman (Breton), Marcel Autret, had been promoted to take his place. Under Aykroyd's directorship he had been chief of the Nutrition Services branch of the Nutrition Division.

When I joined the staff of FAO in January 1961 I was told by Autret that he was going to post me to be FAO adviser on Nutrition to UNICEF in New York, located in the United Nations Headquarters. He told me to find out as much as I could about FAO and the Nutrition Division programmes and activities from the different branch chiefs and also what co-operation they had with UNICEF at that time. He considered me a good candidate for this liaison work because I had had so much experience in the 'bush' in Nigeria working with rural peoples.

A study of the constitution of FAO showed it to have the following objectives — to raise levels of nutrition and standards of living of the world's population; to secure improvements in the efficiency of the production and distribution of all food and agricultural products and to better the conditions of rural populations, thus contributing to the expansion of world economy and 'ensuring man's rights to freedom from hunger'.

In his foreword to the Report of the World Food Congress (FAO, 1963) Dr Sen, then Director General of FAO, stressed that 'the task of abolishing hunger and malnutrition cannot be solved except by a total worldwide effort *in which the governments and the people co-operate*' (the italics are mine). Aykroyd had been a good administrator working in a systematic way and willing to operate within his divisional budget. He had tried to enlist the co-operation of governments and people, first by organising regional conferences in Latin America then in the Indian subcontinent, in the Far East, Indonesia, and in Africa. At these meetings national government representatives and local nutritionists were able to meet the staff of the Nutrition Division and discuss what were the regional and national food and nutrition problems. This was good for both sides of the local and international personnel. He was responsible for starting a series of committees of specialists to prepare reports on man's 'calorie' requirements (1950 and 1957) and on 'protein' requirements (1957). When WHO was founded two years after FAO, Aykroyd bred close co-operation between the WHO Nutrition United directed by Dr R. C. Burgess (Jim) and FAO's Nutrition Division. Aykroyd also stimulated the publication of many monographs known as 'FAO Nutritional Studies' on a variety of subjects such as *Rice and Rice Diets* (1948), *Food Composition Tables for International Use* (1949), *Dietary Surveys: Their Techniques and Interpretation* (1949), *Teaching Better Nutrition* (1950), *School Feeding: its Contribution to Child Nutrition* (1953), *Food Composition Tables — Minerals and Vitamins for International Use* (1954) and others.

Marcel Autret's approach to the administration and technical planning programme of the Nutrition Division was entirely different to that of Wallace Aykroyd. He was more an interagency politician than a technician. His methods of administration and programme preparation were much less systematic and contained less forethought than had those of Aykroyd — volatile in the 'flighty' sense, and opportunistic are good ways of describing his approach. Thus he found it difficult to harness his idea to his budget and was for ever seeking sources to fund the 'projects' he thought had priority at a given time and he persuaded some others of his staff, inexperienced in international affairs, to support them. He did not really understand the importance of obtaining the true backing of the governments of developing countries to support food and nutrition 'programmes' in their countries. The reason was that he could persuade a government to make a request for a specific project which appealed to him and have it financed by the UN Special Fund or, much oftener, by UNICEF. A series of activities conducted in an isolated village or small town in a given country, where school feeding, combined with nutrition education and some elements of home economics and infant care, the whole being called an 'applied nutrition project', was fascinating to UNICEF. The care of mothers, infants and young children excluded care of the family as a complete entity.

DEVELOPING PERSONAL ROOTS IN ENGLAND

The Technical Assistance Board of the UN could be persuaded to fund so-called 'experts' in the field of nutrition, almost all from developed countries with little experience of work in tropical countries and all without any knowledge of public health in relation to nutrition in such developing countries.

The time I spent in Rome from January to early April 1961 gave me the feeling of a lack of cohesion between the different branches of the Nutrition Division. The Nutrition Services Branch, with some co-operation from Home Economics, were dealing with applied nutrition projects (ANPs) or school feeding projects combined with nutrition education. The Food Processing and Preservation Branch were starting to consider the question of food additives and were interested in the development of protein-rich foods made from soya beans in the Far East and from fish in Chile, the latter being conducted in conjunction with UNICEF. This branch was uninterested in the ARLAC project developed in Nigeria. It seemed to me that Autret, as Director, was acting as if he was still chief of the Nutrition Service Branch.

It was made clear to me that my job in New York with UNICEF would be to support Autret's views and support the Nutrition Services Branch approach as highest priority.

In the initial post-war period the UNO developed a fund to administer activities designed to ameliorate the lot of children, in developed and developing countries, whose welfare was put at risk by that conflict because of pestilence, food shortages or socio-economic disturbances of various sorts. This emergency fund was known as the UN International Children's Emergency Fund, which required to support its administration the advice of specialised technical agencies such as WHO, FAO and the ECOSOC Commissions on Social Development, and on the Status of Women. However, this emergency fund was financed by voluntary subscriptions from governments, industrials and by advertisement and the sale of greetings cards, etc. Thus, in common with charitable funds, such as OXFAM, CARE, Save the Children and others it should be careful to put its funds to the best practical use and not to spend too much, as a percentage of its overall reserve, upon staff, administration and maintenance, or upon regional and country representatives offices in developing areas of the world. UNICEF, by its terms of references, and as a non-technical organ of the UN, should rely upon UN

Specialised Agencies such as FAO and WHO and upon ECOSOC Commissions such as those on Social Development or the Status of Women for technical advice upon project developments. As the years went by UNICEF, instead of being a temporary emergency fund, dropped the term 'emergency' from its title and, by exerting influence upon the UN, became a permanent organ of that organisation.

Having acquired this overall picture of FAO and of the interrelationship of UNICEF with the specialised agencies and its status in the UNO, I set out from Rome on 4 April 1961 to advise UNICEF upon any projects which they had been asked for financial support by UN member governments, within the Nutrition Division of FAO's field of competence, about which I admit I was still uncertain.

In the event I found the months I spent with UNICEF to be very boring but I had the compensation in having Mary and the children with me in New York from time to time — Mary most of the time, Diana for summer and Christmas holidays 1961/62 and Christopher for a long summer vacation from Edinburgh University in 1961. He had fixed up with the Shell Oil Company, through the good offices of Douglas Bader and Robert Cain, both of whom we had met for the first time in Lagos, to join the staff of that enormous company provided he acquired a degree in chemical engineering.

He had just finished his first year at the university when he flew out by himself to join me, a week before Mary and Diana followed him. He was quite sure he had failed his exams in maths and organic chemistry and he was unwilling to continue with the idea of joining Shell. We had a talk about an alternative future for him and within a few days he decided he would like to join Barclays Bank Ltd., Dominions, Colonial and Overseas so that he would 'be able to see the world'. I told him he would have to make his peace with his Shell sponsors, and find others to recommend him for a Barclays DCO appointment. During the course of the summer holiday he had achieved both these objectives. When he returned to UK on 7 October he spent some months living in Dorset and working in the Poole branch of Barclays Bank. While he was there he heard that he had passed his first year university exams but decided to go on with the bank notwithstanding the results. He was then posted to Manchester for a year to be trained for service overseas. Thereafter he served in the Bahamas, London, Zambia, and the New Hebrides (now Vanuatu), and has recently worked at the London headquarters of Barclays International, now fused with the UK Barclays Ltd. as Barclays Bank plc.

It was good to have Mary and both children for that summer holiday. While I was tied up in the UN building most days they got around Manhattan seeing the sights from the Statue of Liberty to the Bronx Zoo and places of interest in between. We flew for the September Labor Day weekend to Buffalo and met my sister Susan and her husband Allan Hally at our hotel before going over into Canada with them to see the Niagara Falls. They returned to Toronto where he lived and worked at that time. We were also taken to the Sabins' country house at Monterey, Massachusetts for a weekend's boating and sailing on a nearby lake. During the same trip we visited the Tanglewood Musical Festival ground — an impressive place but no music for us to see and hear.

Diana flew back to school at Melverley in Wimborne, Dorset, met by the husband of the headmistress at Heathrow on 19 September 1961. For all the years we were abroad until she left school he ferried her and other 'overseas' girls to the airport or back from it. She returned to New York for the Christmas holidays from 14 December 61 until 16 January 1962. Like her brother she has travelled widely. After marrying a local man she lived in Papua, New Guinea, and the Middle East, but has now returned to Dorset.

Overall, our life was very hectic in Manhattan. Many of our friends from UK visited, including my mother, all our friends from Nigerian days came to see us if they were passing through New York.

Return to Rome

In May '62 my secretary told me that there were rumours afoot that I would have to return to Rome soon as a permanent posting. I had hinted that I did not like the day-to-day work with UNICEF and would be glad to be posted to Rome. I was looking forward to an Indian and Far Eastern tour which was arranged for the autumn of 1962. But UNICEF was not happy about having an absentee FAO Nutrition Adviser, and Autret had managed to have a post of Assistant to the Director established in the Nutrition Division of FAO which he wanted me to fill.

On 8 June Autret came over to New York for a meeting of the UNICEF Executive Board. He had dinner with us in our apartment and told us we had to be in Rome by 15 July.

Then a hectic rush began. My uncle and aunt, Sir Landsborough and Lady Thomson, turned up in New York in the *Mauritania* for a few days. Mary met them and we got them rooms in the Beekman Towers Hotel. In the next ten days there was a UN reception for the US Mission; a reception by the German Amabassdor to the UN; dinner at home for Autret; a buffet dinner with Sylvia and Joe Orr for Dr B. R. Sen, DG, FAO, and a dinner with the staff of the UN Bureau of Social Services. The UNICEF staff gave me a party in the office.

On 4 July 1962 (Independence Day) we had tickets for a meeting at Independence Hall and saw President John F. Kennedy arrive by helicopter and saw him address the Governors of each and every State of the Union. On 5 July we returned by train to New York and Mary had the apartment packed and cleaned ready for the men to collect our crates and other baggage by 10 July. On 11 July we were finally airborne in an Alitalia Super DC8 and arrived in Rome on Thursday, 12 July 1962. Mario de Crascenzo from the Nutrition Division met us at Leonardo da Vinci airport and drove us to the Pensione Gasser, just off the Piazza Barberini, our normal stopping place for many years in the Eternal City when travelling between Nigeria and UK.

We bathed and rested for the remainder of that day, and the next day, the 14 July 1962, we saw four apartments from a list provided by FAO but none of them were satisfactory. On the 15th (Sunday) we went to see an apartment owned by one of the Gasser sons (Peter) which Signora Gasser had told us would be free of its present Colombian occupants in ten days. Meanwhile we could stay on in the pensione. This ground-floor apartment, with a tiny garden in front, was 32 Via dei Monti Parioli, No. 2, in a beautiful part of the city and was our Roman home from July 1962 until July 1973.

So between 8 June, when told by Autret in New York of my posting to Rome. and 14 July 1962, I had finished my business with UNICEF, Mary had cleared up our apartment at 330 E. 63rd Street, we had arrived in Rome, found ourselves a permanent

DEVELOPING PERSONAL ROOTS IN ENGLAND

residence there and I was ready to start work at FAO HQ as Assistant Director of the Nutrition Division on 15 July according to plan.

Diana arrived on 21 July and on 3 August Christopher came out for his holiday from the bank. On 28 August our luggage arrived from New York with FAO and was sent up to our apartment. Christopher had to return to work on 14 August 1962 and Mary and Diana went back to UK on 17 September, the former to 'Trackway', the latter to Melverley, her school in Wimborne. Mary and Diana had got our Monte Parioli apartment well cleaned, curtained and furbished and we had taken on an apartment at San Felice Circeo and furnished it by the time they left for UK.

I had to fly to Hyderabad, South India, to participate in a UNICEF India and Far East regional meeting from 12-15 October 1962 though the planned conference had been abandoned. I returned to London on 16 October, took delivery of a Humber Super Snipe car from Rootes Cars in West Halkin Street, and drove down to Trackway in it. On 20 October Mary and I flew with this car from Hurn Airport, four miles from Trackway, to Cherbourg and Caen (service for the new car), Moulins night stop, the Mont Cenis Pass to Susa (night stop), Turin, Genoa to Pisa (night stop) to Monte Parioli, reaching there at 4 p.m. on 24 October 1962 to start off my job again as Assistant to the Director of Nutrition Division.

The Headquarters of the Food and Agricultural Organisation of the United Nations (FAO)
The original functions of FAO are set out in the memorial tablet at the Chateau Frontenal in Quebec, Canada, as follows:

'In this building, 16th October 1945, representatives of forty-five nations met and established the Food and Agriculture Organisation, first of the New United Nations Agencies. Thus for the first time nations organised to raise levels of nutrition and to improve production and distribution of food and agricultural products.'

The primary function of FAO, therefore, was to raise the levels of nutrition of the peoples of the world.

The organisation became operational early in 1946 with a comparatively small staff in modest accommodation on New Hampshire Avenue, Washington DC, USA. When I returned to Rome from New York in 1962 its headquarters was in a vast marble building which Mussolini had built to be his Colonial Office, but which had never been occupied. It was wonderfully situated between the Circus Maximus and the Terme di Caracalla (Hot Baths of Caracalla) at the bottom of the fine Via di San Gregorio which leads up between the Palatine and Coelian hills, to the triumphal Arch of Constantine and the Colosseum.

At the end of 1960, when I joined the staff of FAO, the directorial, professional and general service staff (administrative, personal assistants, secretaries, stenographers etc., but not including cleaners, electricians, mechanics and other black-coated personnel) amounted to around 1,500; in 1970 this figure had risen to approximately 3,600 of which only 100 (2.5 per cent) were in the Nutrition Division. Between 1962 and 1970 a completely new block had been added to the original building and by 1973, when I retired from the organisation, yet another block had been completed and was in course of being occupied.

Member governments were entitled to be represented on the professional staff in proportion to the amount of money they contributed to FAO. The only country which was under-represented on this basis was the USA which provided a very large percentage of the organisation's overall budget. The professional calibre of the staff therefore varied considerably, depending largely upon the countries from which individuals were recruited. However, it did not necessarily follow that an individual from a small underdeveloped country was also always of poorer professional material than some of those recruited from developed countries like France, UK, Germany or the USA. From whatever country some of the staff did not pull their weight as well as they should have done according to their paper qualifications. Once appointed a member of the professional or general service staff it was very difficult to get rid of them, only on grounds of poor performance.

The building being a very dominant one in a very historic part of Rome was passed by tourist buses many times daily on their way to places such as the Circus Maximus and Baths of Caracalla. A stock joke of the couriers in such conducted tours, when asked how many people worked in the building was to answer 'about 10 per cent'. After I got to know how things really went inside the building I would estimate the best answer in 1970 would have been 'about 80 per cent of the professional and general service staff which totals about 3,600'.

The organisation was known to all Romans and they all knew where its headquarters was situated.

CASUALTIES ADMITTED TO 19 (GUARDS) LIGHT FIELD AMBULANCE
JULY 1944 to MAY 1945

Period	Locations	Battle Cas.*	Battle Accid.†	Exhaustion	Sick‡	POWs	Civilians	Total
1944 July-Sept. (92 days)	Normandy to Nijmegan	1141	187	104	403	154 (all casualties)	25 (all casualties)	2014
October-December (92 days)	Sittard Galeen St Troud	131	167	13	457	15	23	806
1945 January-March (90 days)	Clearing Reichswald and Rhine Crossings	190	89	16	364	53	5	717
April-8 May (38 days)	Across Rhine to Stade and Cuxhaven	409	100	20	221	101	15	866
Total: July 1944-8 May 1945 (312 days)	Normandy to Cuxhaven	1871 (15% officers 85% ORs)	543 (3% officers 97% ORs)	153 (2% officers 98% ORs)	1445 (4% officers 96% ORs)	323 (all)	68 (all)	4403

* Wounds inflicted by enemy action by gunshot, shells, mortars, grenades and aerial bombs.
† Wounds inflicted by accidental use of weapons or by faulty equipment, e.g. premature shell bursts.
‡ Mainly respiratory tract infections, skin and subcutaneous tissue infections, e.g. boils, digestive tract troubles, varicose veins. Only 6% of all sickness due to venereal disease. cf. 29% of respiratory infections.